Future Imperfect?

Report of the King's Fund Care and Support Inquiry

Melanie Henwood

King's Fund

Published by
King's Fund Publishing
11–13 Cavendish Square
London W1G 0AN

© King's Fund 2001

First published 2001

ISBN 1 85717 450 X

A CIP catalogue record for this book is available from the British Library

Available from:
King's Fund Bookshop
11–13 Cavendish Square
LONDON
W1G 0AN

Tel: 020 7307 2591
Fax: 020 7307 2801

Printed and bound in Great Britain

Cover illustration: creativ collection

Contents

Acknowledgements

Foreword

Executive summary

Acknowledgements

Many people have contributed to the work of the King's Fund Care and Support Inquiry. We are especially grateful to the King's Fund Grants Committee for financing the Inquiry and to Sue Lloyd-Evelyn and Susan Hodge of the King's Fund for their administrative support. Our thanks also go to Christy Billings for background research, to Francis McGlone for help with consultation with service users, and to Adelina Comas-Herrera, Tihana Matosevic and Jeremy Kendall of the Personal Social Services Research Unit at the London School of Economics, for providing quantitative background analysis. We are also grateful to several colleagues for their constructive comments on earlier drafts of the document.

Finally, and most importantly, we are indebted to the many individuals and organisations who took the time to share their perspectives and experiences with us, in written submissions to the Inquiry, in discussions with the Committee, and in consultative meetings.

Foreword

The relationship between the one million people providing care and support services and the many millions of people using those services lies at the heart of this report, just as it is at the heart of health and social care. The quality of care provided is critical for the health, well-being and quality of life, of elderly people, people with a range of disabilities, as well as people with mental health needs, problems of drug or alcohol abuse, or multiple other needs.

In the course of the Inquiry, we were repeatedly struck by the commitment shown to improving the quality of this care. We heard of local innovative and imaginative schemes that harnessed the good will within communities to create a dynamic and caring service. We also heard of a panoply of statutory initiatives designed to improve the quality of care, using regulation and registration, training and funding as levers to improve services.

And yet this Inquiry has also heard a very different story. We have heard from practitioners and policy-makers of purchasing practices that seem to favour inflexible and remote service providers. We have heard about cost management techniques that result in a reduction in the quality of care, and regulatory systems that overlap and contradict each other. We have heard about ambitious training schemes that are still not meeting the needs of people providing this care and support. Most worryingly of all, we have heard – repeatedly – of the difficulty of recruiting and retaining employees who can bring the right commitment, enthusiasm and care to this crucial work.

None of this is new. But in today's context it tells an alarming story. The numbers of people requiring such support, and the complexity of their needs, will increase dramatically. More and more of them will receive care and support in their own homes. And in a booming economy, there is a real fear that people will not choose the jobs that provide the vital care and support they need.

Our recommendations are simple, but they are not simplistic. They warn that, unless we can as a society acknowledge the central importance of this work, we are taking enormous risks both now and in the future. They stress that all our systems and procedures need to concentrate on the vital importance of this relationship between the individual needing care, and the individual giving it. They emphasise the importance of the community in generating support for this work. And most importantly, they argue that we need to restore the esteem and standing of the people doing this vital work. To do this costs money. Failure to do so will cost very much more in the long term if we fail to help people to lead satisfying, full and happy lives in their own homes or in residential care.

My grateful thanks to Melanie Henwood for drawing together the many discussions that have informed our work and to all members of the Inquiry team for their commitment and hard work. Thank you also to all those who made time to share with us their experience and perspectives, and guided our understanding. They will have contributed to reshaping the future quality of care and support which, although still imperfect, has potential for major improvement.

Julia Unwin

Executive summary

Raising the quality of care and support services is increasingly a focus of concern and of policy initiatives to drive up standards. The Care Standards Act (2000) represents a watershed in such developments, and has the potential over time to bring about radical change. However, there can be no room for complacency, and the King's Fund Inquiry into the Quality of Care and Support was established to investigate whether the policy framework *will* produce the intended results, and to consider what further strategies might be necessary to ensure that good quality and responsive services are not simply restricted to pockets of good practice.

There are many hazards and pitfalls in the way of fulfilling the ambitions and potential of the Care Standards Act. Overcoming these will demand both immediate and long-term action, and failure to address this could be catastrophic. Not only would major opportunities be lost, but the increasing complexity of a changing environment, the rising demographic pressure of an ageing population, and the general shortage of a skilled and committed labour force, signals a developing crisis in care. This crisis can only be averted by a coherent and integrated strategy that bridges many central and local departments and agencies.

The Inquiry examined the quality of physical, practical and emotional support to adults who need help for the following reasons:

- frailty in old age
- mental health problems
- physical disabilities
- chronic illness
- learning disabilities
- other needs associated with drug and alcohol misuse and homelessness.

Evidence was gathered from invited written submissions, discussions with key 'witnesses' and consultative meetings with service users and with carers. Although there were examples of good and innovative practice, the experience of many people was of poor services.

Health and social care services are often the focus of negative comments and criticisms, much of which is unhelpful and further depresses staff morale. The purpose of this report is *not* to attack the million or so staff (and countless volunteers) committed to providing high-quality services, but to consider the underlying causes of poor quality and to offer constructive ways forward.

Analysis of the submissions to the Inquiry and of discussions with both individuals and groups identified a number of recurring themes. A striking consensus emerged and the key themes transcended differences that might have been expected between different groups. They included:

- cost and quality
- skills and values of staff
- staffing recruitment and retention
- regulation and training
- management development.

In identifying failings and shortcomings in service quality, the Inquiry recognises that there *have* been considerable improvements, and has not fallen into the trap of false nostalgia for a past 'golden age'. However, we conclude that continued improvement will not occur on the scale needed without urgent attention to a challenging agenda. With this in mind, the following conclusions and recommendations are highlighted by the Inquiry.

Investment

It is an inescapable conclusion that the care sector is under-resourced. Unless this is addressed, it will be impossible to raise the quality of care significantly.

We urge the Government to recognise the significant under-investment in care and support services, and to commit itself to making good the

substantial shortfalls that have occurred year on year. We believe that the order of investment required is likely to be *at least the same* as that being injected into the NHS, i.e. a growth of approximately half in cash terms, and one-third in real terms in just five years. Without such investment, care and support services will be struggling to stand still. They will be unable to address the major improvements needed in quality or to meet the additional requirements of new national standards.

Choice and control

Many service users have no significant choice or control over the services they receive. Real choice and control requires a shift in power relationships from the service purchasers and providers to the service users, while the aim of services should be to help individuals achieve their goals. There *are* good services which do just this. However, too often, service users experience a lack of choice over how, and when, services are delivered, and are expected to fit in with service routines rather than the services being able to respond to individual needs.

The continued development of Direct Payments must be actively promoted. This demands a more proactive approach by the Department of Health, and by local authorities and Care Trusts, in encouraging and supporting take-up of services. This includes giving service users the training and skills they need to become their own service commissioners and care managers. For those service users who do not want to, or are unable to, make use of Direct Payments, other ways (e.g. care planning) must be found of ensuring that real choices and control are built into the use of care and support services. These are vital factors that drive forward service quality.

Cultural responsiveness

Services that are culturally responsive to the diversity of needs of people in black and minority ethnic communities are poorly developed, despite some notable examples of success.

Commissioners of care and support services must encourage the development of a wide range of services to meet the diverse needs of different communities. However, addressing these needs is not something that can be left to specialist services. A key test of mainstream services must be the extent to which they respond appropriately to service users from all cultural and racial backgrounds. We recommend that the Department of Health pays proper attention to addressing cultural responsiveness within the emerging National Minimum Standards agenda. Disseminating information about successful examples of innovative services should be an important early responsibility of the new Social Care Institute for Excellence.

User involvement and empowerment

User involvement and empowerment are words in common use, but too often they are not put into practice. There is also poor understanding of what this concept means at the level of the individual or collectively, e.g. in terms of recognising the diversity of needs or eliminating ageism. Innovative approaches to the genuine involvement of service users in areas such as training and service monitoring have enormous potential to take us beyond rhetoric and tokenism.

We strongly endorse the genuine involvement and empowerment of service users. Users have a vital role to play in areas such as service monitoring and review, and in training staff to better understand users' needs and the principles that should inform care and support. We urge both the Commission for Health Improvement and the Social Care Institute for Excellence: to identify the characteristics of successful examples of such practices and to encourage their widespread adoption.

Cost and quality tensions

Care staff provide a highly valued and essential service for millions of people. The individual commitment and dedication of many staff cannot be faulted. Nonetheless, there is potential for a major deterioration in standards of care. Expenditure constraints have forced local authorities systematically to drive down costs. Although trying to obtain 'Best Value' is a useful concept, it can result in a damaging preoccupation with price at the expense of quality.

We are concerned that the tool of 'Best Value' risks being discredited by the disproportionate emphasis which, in practice, is being laid on driving down costs, at the price of quality. We urge the Department of the Environment, Transport and the Regions (DETR), the Audit Commission and the National Care Standards Commission to review guidance on Best Value to ensure there is adequate recognition that improving service quality is not always synonymous with driving down contract prices.

Commissioning for quality

Most commissioning and contracting of care and support services (both 'in house' and externally) is unsophisticated, poorly related to outcomes and with little regard for levers that might raise service quality.

There is an urgent need to develop commissioning capacity and skills. We propose the Department of Health should issue new guidance to local authorities, Primary Care Trusts and Care Trusts, on best practice in commissioning. This guidance should focus on how best to promote the development of high quality, creative and responsive services. This needs to be matched by strategies to develop and support commissioning capacity and skills, and a clear agenda for the training requirements for commissioning managers.

Changing patterns of service commissioning

Changes in the relationship between health and local authorities, with a move towards closer integration, could do much to overcome old divisions. There are, however, risks in rushing ahead with an untested and insufficiently developed model in which implementation leads policy. The development of new commissioning arrangements, such as those in Care Trusts, must ensure an appropriate level of understanding and knowledge about the needs of service users, by ensuring parity of health and social care interests.

The development of Care Trusts must be approached with caution, rather than 'driven through' as an ideological objective. There are many aspects of the commissioning role in these Trusts that need to be better developed. The Department of Health must take responsibility for appropriate governance arrangements. It must also ensure there is an appropriate level of understanding and knowledge about the needs of service users, by ensuring parity of health and social care interests.

Reviewing the National Vocational Qualification (NVQ)

There is considerable discontent about the NVQ model in care and support. In view of the strong emphasis being placed on the attainment of NVQ within national standards, a major review and overhaul of assessment and verification of NVQ is an urgent priority.

We recommend three complementary actions to address shortcomings with NVQs:

- The Qualifications and Curriculum Authority (QCA), and awarding bodies offering Care NVQs, should undertake an immediate review to determine the consistency of assessment, and take any necessary action arising.

- A review of the National Occupational Standards that provide the content of Care NVQs is underway by TOPSS and Healthwork UK, and due to be completed by 2003. We recommend that as part of the review, work should be undertaken to strengthen assessment requirements and improve consistency.

- Work should be undertaken by TOPSS and Healthwork UK to improve the quality of work-based assessment through better support to line managers undertaking assessment.

Developing skills and competence

The care and support sectors suffer from a tradition of employing unskilled labour. Radical change is needed to transform the sector's image into one that better reflects the reality of the work involved. It is important to build on the wealth of experience of staff and to develop their skills and knowledge appropriately, underpinned at all stages by attention to core underlying values.

We recommend that TOPSS and Healthwork UK urgently progress work to ensure that all training builds on the skills of staff and develops competence on the basis of appropriate qualifications. Equal weight must be given to developing underlying values and attitudes as to the acquisition of practical and technical skills. The identification of various learning routes to qualifications should be a priority.

Supporting the costs of training

For independent providers, the costs of investing in staff training are an important disincentive to providing employees with more than the basic minimum of induction. A range of more creative approaches to supporting the costs of training is required.

Local authorities must work with providers to raise the skills and standards of all care staff. Supporting the costs of training staff to higher standards necessitates that providers are able to reflect the realistic costs of training within their contract prices, and/or that local authorities ensure access to the resources of the Training Support Programme. We also recommend that TOPSS, Healthwork UK and the new Learning and Skills Council should consider financial incentives for employers and employees to train and achieve higher level skills by means of:

- **Individual Learning Accounts (ILAs) enhanced through additional contributions from employers and/or regulators**
- **training loans – including transferable training loans – targeted especially at independent sector providers.**

We recommend piloting of these methods as a matter of urgency.

Recruitment and retention

The recruitment and retention of staff in care and support services is a major and growing challenge that demands imaginative and creative solutions to avoid a crisis. Improved pay and conditions must be at the heart of the solution, while other ways of raising the status of care workers are also crucial.

> **We urge the Department of Health to be imaginative and flexible in developing strategies to raise the status and image of the care and support sector, and to recognise that these must go far beyond reforming social work training. At the heart of this must be realistic and appropriate remuneration for highly demanding work, improved conditions of employment and career prospects. Other approaches to enhancing the status of care workers should be piloted, including exploring the effects of different titles (such as 'personal care assistants' or 'community care workers') which better reflect the skilled and valued work that care workers undertake. Other experimentation with changing the pattern of incentives might focus on extending 'key worker' status to care and support workers in localities where there are particular problems with recruitment and retention.**

Sharing and disseminating strategies

The Department of Health should take the lead in promoting strategies to improve recruitment and retention. Successful approaches in both the health and care sectors should be widely shared.

> **We recommend that the remit of the National Workforce Development Board in the Department of Health should be a wide one that goes beyond health care. This would provide a particular opportunity to address the interdependencies between the health and care employment sectors. The Development Board should take responsibility for identifying and disseminating examples of successful recruitment and retention strategies in health and care which might be more widely adopted.**

Encompassing volunteers

The role of volunteers alongside paid staff is a vital one that has to be supported and encouraged. However, this reserve army should not be treated as a ready solution to the problems of labour supply and a cheap substitute for a skilled and trained workforce.

Measures to encourage volunteering in health and care need to understand the complementary role which volunteers play, and not treat them as substitute labour. The Government's enthusiasm for volunteers, and its emphasis on the responsibilities of everyone in a civic society must be matched by the development of a Charter for volunteers which addresses their rights, as well as those of the people they support. The need for adequate quality safeguards to check the suitability of volunteers is vital, and the operation of the new Criminal Records Bureau will need to be carefully monitored to ensure that it is meeting disclosure requirements.

Intelligent regulation

New regulatory structures and mechanisms introduce an opportunity to transform the shape of social care. However, there are complexities to be overcome and approaches need to be 'intelligent' and avoid the pitfalls of over-bureaucracy. The focus on qualification as the sole path to registration is misplaced and will result in a considerable delay before the aspirations of the Care Standards Act can be fully realised.

We recommend that the General Social Care Council should adopt a revised timetable for the registration of care workers that does not rely solely on registration based on qualification. An interim register should also be developed which includes all unqualified social care workers employed by local authorities and in the independent sector, and establishes target dates for their full registration on the basis of qualification. We also urge that in bringing forward proposals for the regulation of health support workers, the Department of Health is mindful of the opportunity for – and importance of – developing a coherent

approach between the remit of the General Social Care Council and whatever additional regulatory body is given responsibility in the health field.

Management development

Management infrastructure and capacity in social care have been key casualties of financial restraint. Investment in the care sector will not be enough to raise standards unless there is a parallel emphasis on how resources are used and what is generated.

There is an undeniable need to invest in the development of management and leadership skills across the public and independent sectors of care and support. We recommend the urgent development of appropriate management training as a priority. The Department of Health should take the lead in supporting management development at all organisational levels. Requirements to obtain management qualifications and skills must be matched by opportunities to do so, and there may be scope for building on the foundation of Individual Learning Accounts to encourage take-up by employees and employers alike.

A failure to tackle this demanding agenda would be shortsighted, while for the millions of current and future service users and their carers, it could indeed be catastrophic. The future will always be imperfect, but we believe that the solutions we are offering have the potential to transform the quality of care and support services.

1   Introduction

1.1   The Care and Support Inquiry was established by the King's Fund in Spring 2000. Julia Unwin was appointed as Chair of the Inquiry, and Melanie Henwood was commissioned to provide the secretariat. A Committee was established and met eight times between May 2000 and March 2001. The Inquiry was charged with examining the quality of physical, practical or emotional support given to adults needing help because of:

- frailty in old age
- mental health problems
- physical disabilities
- chronic illness
- learning disabilities
- acquired immune deficiency syndrome (AIDS) or human immunodeficiency virus (HIV) infection
- drug or alcohol dependency
- homelessness.

Our focus was principally on England. It also included relevant issues within other regions of the UK or, when appropriate, further afield

1.2   The definition of 'physical, practical, or emotional support' as the focus of the Inquiry opens a window on a wide range of services and different types of care and support workers. This includes staff involved in *personal care*, who are variously known as care assistants/health care assistants, home carers, or care staff. Personal care includes help with self-care and activities of daily living, such as washing and dressing, getting in and out of bed, toileting, bathing, feeding, etc. It also includes tasks and interventions closer to nursing care, including help with medication, catheter care, etc. There is often an overlap between staff working in health and social care settings, both of whom may be providing personal care. We did not, however, focus on other types of *health* support workers, e.g. auxiliary nurses, physiotherapy assistants, therapy assistants, theatre assistants, etc. A separate review of the roles, functions and responsibilities of these workers, and recommendations for appropriate regulation, has already been undertaken by De Montford University for the Department of Health, and we saw no value in simply replicating this analysis. The findings from the De Montford review had not been published during the course of our Inquiry.

1.3   The Inquiry was concerned not only with 'hands-on' care, but also with support provided to assist people in participating in daily life. This includes providing extra support to people with a mental health problem or a learning disability, for example, in accessing further education and training; obtaining and holding down a job; participating in leisure activities; coping with personal financial matters; or finding their way through the system of services and bureaucracies. The staff involved in such work are usually known as support workers, but may have other titles, such as job coaches or advocates.

1.4   Care and support workers are employed by a range of public, private and voluntary organisations, such as local authorities, the NHS, and independent sector agencies. They work in a variety of settings, including hospitals, hospices, care homes, community facilities, sheltered housing, and people's own homes. Some workers, usually known as personal assistants, are employed directly by individual service users on a one-to-one basis.

1.5   The establishment of the Inquiry reflected a growing concern over the poor quality of services, and took place at a time when the quality of health and care was increasingly on the policy agenda. This is reflected, for example, in the establishment of National Service Frameworks for key client groups and by the development of a range of structures and mechanisms for improving standards. Of most direct relevance is the Care Standards Act (2000), which has introduced a new regulatory framework for social care, aimed at improving public protection and increasing standards in the workforce and service delivery. Some might ask whether this Inquiry has been timely. They may query whether the Inquiry is being premature in trying to make judgements at a time of change when new regulations are coming into force. On the contrary, we believe that this is *precisely the right time* to examine the issues involved in greater detail, and to ask whether the changes being put in place to raise quality will be sufficient, and if not, to explore what else must be addressed.

1.6   Despite examples of innovative practice, too often services fail to measure up and there are instances of neglect and failure. However, there are wider concerns about the perceived failure of services to provide the type of care and support that promotes independence and inclusion, and enables people to take part in ordinary life. The reasons for these failings were important issues for the Inquiry. It is easy to criticise service shortcomings, but more demanding to try and understand the causes of such problems and to find practical ways of overcoming them. The Inquiry therefore addressed several issues:

- the identification and exploration of problems in the quality of care and support services
- the causes of these problems and the complexity of different causal factors and influences
- an understanding of the characteristics of innovative practice and the factors most likely to contribute to its development
- an assessment of the adequacy and proportionality of the current and developing policy response
- conclusions and recommendations for the way forward.

1.7   In addressing this wide agenda, the Committee sought to hear the voices of the many different individuals and organisations involved. A review of the relevant literature and research material was undertaken and continued to evolve throughout the life of the Inquiry. Additional small pieces of research were commissioned as necessary to contribute to the knowledge base and inform analysis of the issues. Written submissions were invited and more than 120 documents were received. The Committee used several meetings to explore specific issues in greater depth with 'witnesses' invited to share their expertise and insights. Other methods of consultation were also used to ensure the representation of the voices of service users and carers who might otherwise be overlooked by the more formal approaches to evidence gathering.

1.8   The subject of the Inquiry is one on which opinions and passions run high. It is also an area in which there are tensions between different interests. Our conclusions and recommendations are concerned with bringing about genuine change and lasting improvement. Their achievement will be demanding and will require fundamental shifts in attitudes and values, at all levels of society. A failure to address this agenda now would be a failure not only for the present generation, but for those to come. The forces behind the steady build-up of pressure at the current time are likely to become even more intense, and to force a genuine crisis in the care and support services, if this does not take place.

Julia Unwin

Julia Unwin OBE
(Chair of Inquiry)

Ziggi Alexander
Chair, CCETSW and TOPSS
UK Partnership

Melvyn Carlowe OBE
Former Chief Executive, Jewish Care,
Voluntary Sector Consultant

Cliff Prior
Chief Executive
National Schizophrenia Fellowship

Rodney Bickerstaffe
President, National Pensioners
Convention, and Former General
Secretary, UNISON

Frances Hasler
Co-Director,
National Centre for Independent Living

Janice Robinson
Director, Health and Social Care
Programme, King's Fund

Clive Bowman FRCP
Physician and Gerontologist
University of Bristol, and
Medical Director, BUPA
Care Services

Melanie Henwood
Secretary and Rapporteur to Inquiry,
Independent Health and Social Care
Consultant

Chris Vellenoweth
Independent Adviser,
Health Policy

Catherine McLoughlin CBE
Chair, St George's Healthcare NHS Trust

Lydia Yee
Carer and Independent
Consultant

2 Background and context

2.1 The policy agenda in social care, the health service and other key public services, is increasingly characterised by aspirations to improve quality. Government Ministers repeatedly proclaim the need for more accessible, consistent and convenient services which protect those they care for, while also offering greater choice, control and flexibility to service users. Such developments are to be welcomed. However, the attainment of these objectives will take time. The need for a new vision and culture to transform services is recognised in policy statements. However, critical questions need to be asked about the process for bringing about this transformation, and the likely timescale for its completion.

2.2 'Quality' is not an objective or absolute standard. In general, definitions of quality vary not only over time (typically, aspirations and expectations rise year-on-year), but between individuals, people of different ages and socio-economic groups. Quality tends to convey different meanings in private and public sectors. In the public sector, it has typically been associated with services that are acceptable, adequate, or 'good enough' rather than with excellence. The poor quality of services becomes newsworthy only in the event of a scandal or tragedy. The history of the post-war Welfare State is one of progress and development, punctuated by frequent inquiries into abuse and neglect, both in institutional and other settings. Much of the concern has focused on the general welfare of children, particularly the repeated, devastating failures of the child protection system. Although child welfare is vitally important, the focus of our Inquiry is on adult service users.

2.3 Criticisms of social services are widespread and directed at several issues. As the Department of Health itself acknowledges, some of this criticism is misplaced. Some of it, however, is not.[1] The criticisms can be summarised as follows:

- Services are not of the highest quality.

- Staff are often either not trained or inadequately trained.

- Services are often bureaucratic and inflexible.

- Access to services can be problematic.

- Health and social services do not always work in partnership.

- Services are geographically inconsistent and variable.[2]

2.4   An understanding of the scale and significance of the care and support sector is a prerequisite for any investigation into the problems and challenges to be addressed. The Royal Commission on Long Term Care, which reported in 1999,[3] also set out to establish a profile of the sector. It immediately encountered problems because there was no central database, and it had difficulties in accounting for expenditures listed under different budgetary headings. Using a model developed by the Personal Social Services Research Unit (PSSRU), the Commission estimated the total cost of long-term care for the UK at £11.1 billion in 1996. This included expenditure by the NHS and social services, but not for general practitioner (GP) services, housing, leisure services or unpaid care. Similarly, the estimate included the accommodation costs of hospitals and care homes, but *not* the housing costs for people living in ordinary or sheltered housing.[4]

2.5   The difficulties inherent in the data are apparent. It is also clear that the size of the long-term care sector (and of the wider field of care and support) is considerable. In seeking to develop a profile of the health and care sector, the Inquiry also encountered problems with the quality and availability of data. To overcome this, the Inquiry commissioned a background analysis from the PSSRU (see Appendix 1). Some of the key facts and figures of the analysis are highlighted below.

2.6   The profile of the sector needs to be understood within the context of the development of 'the mixed economy of care'. There has been a change in the role of the local authority from that of being primarily a service provider to being a commissioner and organiser of services, with a reduced role in direct provision. This development was a direct result of the community care reforms introduced by the 1990 NHS and Community Care Act, based on the Griffiths report of 1988.[5] The 1990 Act required local authorities to encourage the development of non-statutory service providers. Griffiths and the subsequent White Paper, *Caring for People*,[6] had argued that the promotion of the independent sector, including both private and voluntary services, would produce greater choice, innovation, and flexibility in services, and improved value for money through competition. The resulting growth of the independent sector as the major provider of care and support has been dramatic. In the case of domiciliary care, virtually all the growth in this sector has taken place since the early 1990s.

Mapping the sectors

2.7   Below we highlight some of the key facts and figures that describe the scale of the health and care sectors in terms of the workforce, expenditure, staffing and employment (see Appendix 1 for full details).

- The value of the social care sector in terms of total expenditure across the private and public sectors is considerable. In the year 2000, it is estimated that the value of care for elderly people, chronically ill and physically disabled people in the UK was £13.2 billion, comprising £8.6 billion residential care and £4.6 billion non-residential care.

- The gross expenditure of local authority social services departments on both adult and children's services was £10.8 billion in 1998–99. This indicates a steady growth, from £5.6 billion a decade earlier.

- Expenditure on services for older people accounts for 48 per cent of social services spending. Expenditure on other adult client groups was as follows: 14 per cent on learning disabilities; 7 per cent on people with a physical disability; 5 per cent on people with mental health problems; and 0.6 per cent on HIV infection or AIDS, and drug and alcohol misuse. Only 1.4 per cent of total social services expenditure was committed to service strategy and central development.

- The total value of the UK market in residential/nursing home care in 2000 was estimated at £8.6 billion. In 1988, the public sector provided

52 per cent of the total market value of care; by 2000 this figure had fallen to 22 per cent.

- Gross expenditure, including both public and private expenditure, on non-residential services was estimated at almost £4.6 billion in 1998–99; some £575 million of this was personal expenditure.

- The total number of people employed in social care in England is estimated at between 900,000 and 1.2 million, two-thirds of whom work in the independent sector, mainly in residential homes.

- The estimate of 900,000 is likely to be a conservative figure, which significantly *underestimates* the full size of the social care workforce, the gaps left by specialist surveys may represent an additional 40,000 staff.

- Fourteen per cent (127,000) are home care workers in the independent sector, and 8 per cent (74,000) are local authority home care workers.

- About 54 per cent (487,000) staff are care assistants in independent residential and nursing homes.

- Health care assistants comprise a small proportion (approximately 3 per cent) of the total care workforce.

- There has been an 18 per cent fall in the whole-time equivalent numbers of staff working in local authority residential care in the five years between 1994 and 1999, which probably reflects the increased use of the independent sector. Similar trends are evident in local authority home care services, where the whole-time equivalent workforce has fallen by 20 per cent.

- While there are *fewer* care staff working in local authorities, there have been parallel *increases* in the numbers employed in social services headquarters in central and strategic roles – from 15,000 whole-time equivalents in 1994 to 19,000 by 1999.

2.8   This introductory overview of the economic and financial context of care and support has mapped the key features of the sectors. The sectors are economically significant in size, and are major employers. There has been an increasing shift in the pattern of employment, with reduced importance for the local authority as a direct provider (and hence employer), and an accompanying growth in the contribution of the independent (private and voluntary) sector.

2.9 Most people use care and support services provided by the independent sector, although these are often commissioned through the local authority. Service users are means-tested for these services and are charged by the local authority. There is also a growing area of private funding whereby service users purchase their care directly from independent service providers.

A changing environment

2.10 As well as understanding the overall shape and changing nature of the care sector, the Inquiry needed to place its investigations within the context of a developing and shifting environment (Figure 2.1). In this respect, a number of aspects are particularly important and will be discussed below, such as:

- the policy context
- demographic and social trends
- economic and employment factors.

The policy context

2.11 The policy environment is a complex one. At its heart, are policy developments concerning health and social care that have a direct and immediate impact. Besides these, there are other policy developments, including:

- the modernisation agenda
- housing and urban regeneration
- education and training
- employment.

This section of the report does not attempt to document the minutiae of all of these different aspects, but focuses on those which have a lesser or greater impact in shaping the health and care environment.

Figure 2.1 The external environment influencing the quality of care and support

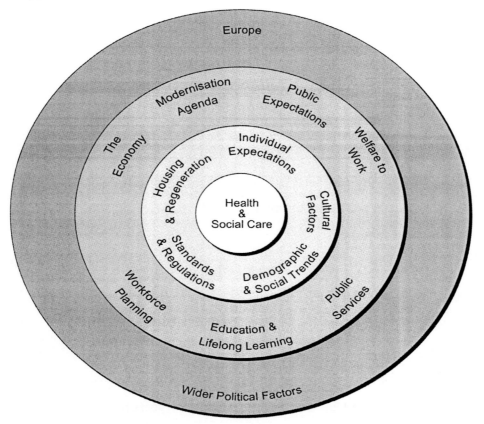

2.12   Part of the reason for outlining the broad nature of this policy environment is because, since taking office in May 1997, the Labour government has increasingly emphasised the need for coherent policy-making and 'joined-up' government, rather than rigid and separatist departmentalism. It is recognised that actions in any one sector will have consequences – expected or unexpected – on other parts of the system. Indeed, the problems of a disjointed approach to policy-making have long been recognised. Various attempts have been made to introduce some degree of co-ordination and coherence, notably the Joint Approaches to Social Policy (JASP) initiative of the Central Policy Review Staff in the mid-1970s.[7] However, since New Labour came to power, there has been renewed interest in such developments, and a greater impetus given to them by the establishment of a Cabinet-level co-ordinator.

Modernising government

2.13   One practical manifestation of the 'joined-up' ideology is the 'modernising government' strategy that extends throughout government departments. This is characterised by an emphasis on several themes, all of which recur in the health and care sector:

- improved policy-making through socially inclusive and evidence-based policies

- more responsive services

- higher quality services

- modern public sector management.

2.14   The emergence of social inclusion as a policy objective is a theme that is evident on a number of levels, reflected in the development of the Social Exclusion Unit. 'Social exclusion' refers to a complex interaction of issues. At its core, there is a concern to reduce poverty, as defined in terms of 'low incomes, lack of work, low levels of skills, lack of access to good-quality public services and lack of opportunities to live active and fulfilling lives'.[8] Specific strategies have been developed to tackle certain priorities, such as truancy, teenage pregnancy, rough sleeping, and drug and alcohol misuse. In addition, the broad ethos of promoting social inclusion has been expressed through recent Race Relations legislation and the Human Rights Act (2000).

2.15   The Race Relations (Amendment) Act 2000 needs to be seen in the light of the Macpherson Inquiry[9] into the death of Stephen Lawrence, and its scrutiny of all public services, including their policies, practices and procedures, for indications of institutionalised racism. The Act provides new powers to tackle racism in public authorities by:

- outlawing direct and indirect discrimination in public authority functions

- placing a general duty on public authorities to work towards eliminating unlawful discrimination and to promote equality of opportunity and good relations between different racial groups.

2.16   The Human Rights Act came into force in October 2000. For the first time, UK citizens can seek protection of their rights (under the European Convention on Human Rights) within the UK courts, rather than having to seek redress in Europe. As Britain has long been a signatory to the European Convention, much public practice should be in compliance with the Act. Nonetheless, the Act places a new onus on public authorities (and private bodies contracted by public bodies) to ensure that their policies and practices are in accordance with Human Rights legislation. The Department of Health has issued guidelines on the type of cases that might now be covered by such legislation.[10] It is early days yet, but it is likely that legal challenges will be made on issues with profound implications for care and support services. For example, practices may be challenged that have tended to diminish the rights of people with mental health problems, learning disabilities, or mental incapacity, in favour of the collective rights and safety of society.[11] However, the Act does include exemptions in respect of people judged to have unsound mind.

2.17   Both the Race Relations (Amendment) Act and the Human Rights Act provide a legislative framework that introduces important levers for change. In the health and care sector, their relevance lies in the opportunity for improving service to a range of vulnerable groups, including those in minority communities. They should also improve employment conditions in a sector that employs disproportionately high numbers of employees from black and minority ethnic groups.

Older people

2.18   As we have noted previously, older people are major users of care services. Increasingly, their numeric importance is accompanied by their growing significance as a political force. For some years, gerontologists and policy commentators have talked of the potential of 'grey power' becoming a more important demographic force as the ageing population becomes larger. In contrast to the USA and its 'grey panthers', and several other European countries, pensioner power has been slow in the UK to become organised or influential. However, the confrontation with the National Pensioners Convention lobby at the 2000 Annual Labour Party Conference forced the Government to reconsider its treatment of this numerically significant group, incensed at the minimal £0.75 weekly increase to the State pension. This incident can be seen as a significant benchmark in the growing political force of the older population in the UK.

2.19   The increased attention to older people has been reflected in other policy developments, including concessions over winter fuel payments, free TV licenses for the over-75s, and the new Minimum Income Guarantee, as well as in steps to address age discrimination. The importance of addressing issues for older people in a 'joined-up' fashion has been shown by the establishment of an Inter-Ministerial Group on Older People responsible for co-ordinating issues affecting older people, and by the Better Government for Older People (BGOP) programme established by the Cabinet Office. Twenty-eight BGOP pilot projects were set up to develop more integrated strategies and to engage actively with older people. The most important single message from the BGOP programme, according to its Steering Group, was 'that working together with older people produces better and more effective solutions'.[12] The Government's response to the BGOP programme's recommendations emphasised the twin themes of partnership and innovation, and praised the initiative as 'an excellent example of what can be achieved when national and local government work together with voluntary organisations and other agencies to provide better services for the public'.[13]

Health and care

2.20   As noted earlier, policy in health and social care has had the most direct impact on the territory with which the Inquiry is concerned. The policy emphasis on developing community-based support is long-standing, and has been particularly explicit since publication of the 1989 White Paper, *Caring for People*,[14] and the subsequent community care reforms in 1993. The major objective of policy continues to be promoting community-based alternatives to residential care and enhancing the independence of service users. The 1998 White Paper, *Modernising Social Services*,[15] re-stated such concerns by emphasising the need to 'promote people's independence while treating them with dignity and respect at all times, and protecting their safety'.

2.21 Recently, there has been a slight change in emphasis. It is now recognised that targeting support where need is greatest – at the heart of the *Caring for People* reforms – has meant people are unlikely to receive support until their needs have become intense. Thus, a key component of *Modernising Social Services* has been to encourage a new form of targeting, aimed at directing low-level support to people most 'at risk' of losing their independence. A new three-year grant has recently been introduced to facilitate such support.

2.22 A recurrent theme in New Labour policy has been the search for a 'third way', as an alternative to polarised ideological preferences for or against market solutions. As stated in 1998, in the social services White Paper:

> *The last Government's devotion to privatisation of care provision put dogma before users' interests, and threatened a fragmentation of vital services. But it is also true that the near-monopoly local authority provision that used to be a feature of social care led to a 'one size fits all' approach where users were expected to accommodate themselves to the services that existed. Our third way for social care moves the focus away from who provides the care, and places it firmly on the quality of services experienced by, and outcomes achieved for, individuals and their carers and families.*[16]

2.23 This approach has been reinforced by the development of a 'concordat' between local authorities and private care home providers. It is intended to 'signal the beginning of a new mature relationship between the players, using capacity and resources to best effect, with maximum benefit for patients'.[17]

2.24 The approach of the Labour government to social care has therefore been one of incremental change and continuity rather than revolutionary upheaval.[18] As others have also observed, Labour has not set out to reverse the establishment of the social care market.[19] It has increasingly emphasised collaboration rather than competition. Indeed, the continuation of the market seems assured by an emphasis on pragmatism. As the Secretary of State for Health told the 1999 annual social services conference, 'it is no longer who provides the social care that matters. It is the quality of care that counts'.[20]

Partnerships and Care Trusts

2.25 Just as improved co-ordination of services has been a major and recurrent theme in public policy in general, it has also been important in health and social policy. Since 1997, there has been an increasing emphasis on effective joint working between health and social services, and between these services and the wider corporate local authority agenda. Specific arrangements for improving partnership through a range of new 'flexibilities' were contained in the Health Act (1999), and came into operation in April 2000. The Act removed legal obstacles to joint working by allowing the use of:

- *pooled budgets*, where health and social services put resources into a joint budget to fund a range of local care services
- *lead commissioning*, in which it is agreed that either the local authority, or the health authority/Primary Care Trust takes the lead in commissioning services on behalf of both in order to overcome overlaps and gaps
- *integrated providers*, with local authorities and health authorities merging their services into a single provider.

The publication of the NHS Plan in July 2000 saw the upgrading of these partnership flexibilities from optional to mandatory status,[21] with the Secretary of State announcing that 'we will make it a requirement for these powers to be used in all parts of the country rather than just some. The result will be a new relationship in health and social care'.[22] A key test of these closer working relationships is said to be 'how well they provide older people with improved services'.[23] In particular, there is an emphasis on developing new intermediate care services 'to promote independence and improve quality of care for older people'. By 2003–04, £900 million is to be allocated to these services, which will include:

- rapid-response teams to prevent unnecessary hospital admissions
- intensive rehabilitation services
- recuperation facilities
- one-stop shop services based in the community
- integrated home care teams to support living independently at home.

2.26   The use of the Health Act flexibilities, and new resources to pursue such objectives, could have a major impact in reconfiguring care services. According to the Department of Health, the development of intermediate care services will 'enable increased numbers of older people to maintain independent lives at home', while contributing to the overall efficiency and effectiveness of the health and social care system through 'more effective use of acute capacity'. They will also contribute to the meeting of waiting list targets.[24]

2.27   The NHS Plan also introduced the establishment of new hybrid 'Care Trusts' as the next stage of development of Primary Care Trusts. They will enable closer integration of health and social services through new, single, multi-purpose bodies responsible for all local health and social care:

> *Care Trusts will be able to commission and deliver primary and community health care as well as social care for older people and other client groups ... Care Trusts will usually be established where there is a joint agreement at local level that this model offers the best way to deliver better services.*[25]

2.28 Initially the Secretary of State for Health argued that partnerships – including Care Trusts – could not be viewed as optional developments. Where services were believed to be failing, powers would be taken to force the establishment of integrated arrangements. There is an expectation that *all* adult social care services will be commissioned through Care Trusts within five years.[26] However, during the third reading of the Health and Social Care Bill, prior to the dissolution of Parliament in May 2001, the Government backed down on the issue of compulsory Care Trusts, in response to widespread disquiet from the Association of Directors of Social Services and others. It is likely that the change may prove more apparent than real; while Care Trusts may not be imposed, it is intended that powers to require the use of the Health Act partnership arrangements will remain. The pressure to establish Care Trusts is likely to be inexorable.

2.29 The modernisation agenda was also re-stated in the NHS Plan, which set out a vision 'to offer people fast and convenient care delivered to a consistently high standard. Services will be available when people require them, tailored to their individual needs'.[27] The NHS Plan identified the failings of the health service as being insufficiently responsive to the convenience and concerns of the patient and being essentially a 1940s system operating in a twenty-first century world.

2.30 The specification of national standards in public services is increasingly prominent. As pointed out by Hudson, varying patterns of accountability in the NHS and social services have resulted in different types of relationship between the central and local agencies. However, this distinction is increasingly blurred.[28] Traditionally, the NHS has been directly accountable to the Secretary of State for Health, while social services have been accountable to locally elected councils. In addition, 'while it has been common practice for some time for the Department of Health to set out national targets and other arrangements to be met by the NHS locally, this has not been felt to be appropriate for social services. This is no longer the position'.[29] Instead, the Labour government has introduced a range of national requirements for both services, signalling a move towards what Hudson describes as a 'nationalisation' of local authority social services, characterised by 'an unprecedented degree of central command and surveillance'. Such national requirements are reflected in joint national priorities guidance, and in the development of National Service Frameworks for key client groups and clinical conditions.

2.31   A National Service Framework for mental health was issued in 1999,[30] and one for older people in March 2001.[31] The Framework approach is characterised by:

- specification of national standards, grounded as far as possible on an evidence base
- a statement of what objectives are to be achieved
- clarity about how performance is to be measured.

2.32   Increased centralisation is evident in the establishment of structural mechanisms for quality control and improved consistency, such as the Commission for Health Improvement, the National Institute for Clinical Excellence, and the Social Care Institute for Excellence. These are crucial components of the Government's strategy. The Government sees regulation as the key to improved service quality. The establishment of national standards and service models will provide a framework for setting local service standards and criteria, telling people what to expect, and providing a way of measuring improvement. The creation of the National Care Standards Commission and the General Social Care Council by the Care Standards Act (2000) has provided a new regulatory framework for social care, 'with the aim of improving protection and driving up standards both in the workforce and in service delivery'.[32] The National Care Standards Commission will be responsible for ensuring that all regulated care services are provided to National Minimum Standards, and advising Ministers about the adequacy of those standards. The GSSC will regulate the social care workforce and social work training, 'which will increase the levels of safety offered to service users, their carers and the general public'. The complexity and multilayered nature of the structures being put in place to improve quality are illustrated in Figure 2.2.

2.33   Alongside the complex framework for improving quality that is being established at central level, it is also recognised that much depends on local implementation. The Department of Health has identified a number of essential components for delivering the 'quality strategy' at local level, including:

- 'implementing Best Value, which will drive continuous improvement in the way services are provided by local authorities

- the introduction of a framework to ensure continuous quality improvement, which emphasises the importance of staff development and training together with high standards of practice at all levels

- actively fostering a culture within social services that emphasises Lifelong Learning

- creating a sound evidence base from which to drive service change

- generating and cementing creative partnerships between all sectors and across all fields, to develop innovative and flexible services

- the imaginative use of information technology

- regular and rigorous assessment of local councils' performance in achieving these goals'.[33]

2.34   Whether the quality strategy set out by the Department of Health is adequate or appropriate to deliver the stated objectives of improving consistency, ensuring services are tailored to individual need, and producing a better trained and more confident workforce, are issues to which we return later in Sections 3 and 4 of this report.

2.35   A further major theme that runs through health and care policy is that of user/patient involvement. In recent years, there has been a growing recognition of the importance of not only *informing* service users about services, but of actively engaging them in planning and evaluation processes. For example, the National Priorities Guidance includes the shared objective for health and social care that users and carers should be 'actively involved' in planning services and in tailoring individual packages of care. National surveys of patient and user experience have also been introduced to 'give patients and their carers a voice in shaping the modern and dependable NHS'.[34] More recently, the NHS Plan included proposals for modernising the way patients' views are represented within the NHS through a new Patient Advocacy and Liaison Service (PALS) to be established in every Trust. In addition, there were to be 'other new citizens' empowerment mechanisms', including setting up a Patients' Forum in every NHS Trust and Primary Care Trust, and giving patients direct representation on every Trust board.

2.36   The NHS Plan also contained controversial, and largely unexpected, proposals for the abolition of Community Health Councils (CHCs). During debate of the Bill, Ministers were forced into concessions on new forms of patient representation to satisfy Labour backbenchers and opposition peers. However, with time running out for the Health and Care Bill prior to the dissolution of parliament in May 2001, the proposals on CHCs were withdrawn (although the responsibility to establish an independent patient advocacy service will remain). If returned to power, the Labour government would seek to reintroduce measures to change patient representation within the NHS through patients forums.

2.37   As we emphasised earlier, while the health and care agenda is the most important part of the policy context with which we are concerned, it is by no means the only aspect. We now turn to consider other factors that also influence the actual, or potential, demand for care and support and its supply.

Figure 2.2 Supporting the quality agenda

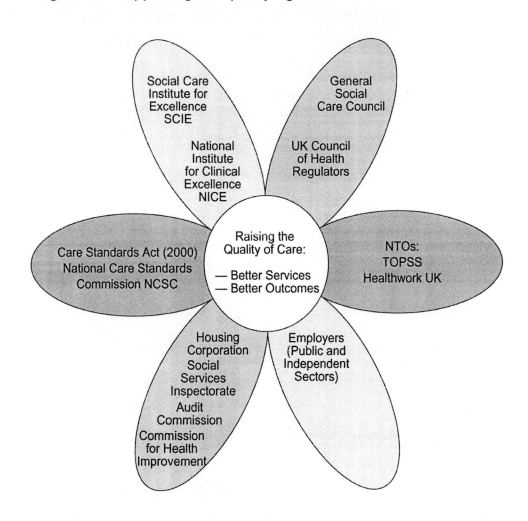

Housing and community care

2.38   Developments in housing and regeneration policy also form an important part of the context to the Inquiry. In particular, these developments affect the capacity of older and disabled people to remain living in their own homes or in supported housing, and to participate fully in local communities. They also influence where, and how, care and support staff perform their work. The Department of Environment and Department of Health issued a joint circular on housing and community care in 1992, which emphasised that housing has an important role to play in community care and is in many ways the key to independent living.[35] The Audit Commission's 1998 analysis of the contribution of housing to community care emphasised both housing and support issues.[36] Whereas the role of housing used to be considered largely in terms of 'special needs housing', there is an increased emphasis on the use of ordinary housing, with suitable adaptations and 'floating' support.

2.39   The Commission estimated that at least 1.3 million tenants and owner occupiers are beneficiaries of housing-related community care services, as provided by council housing departments and through Registered Social Landlords (RSLs). Table 2.1 summarises the types of housing services provided.

2.40   The Audit Commission underlined problems of co-ordination, and despite some evidence of progress and good practice, they painted a picture of 'inadequate identification of needs, inflexible use of stock and insufficient early intervention to prevent vulnerable people reaching crisis point'. Poor collaboration between housing, social services and health authorities was seen as responsible for too many people falling through the net. In particular, for people with mental health problems, the consequence was often that of a 'revolving door' between hospital and home.

2.41   The Audit Commission found housing authorities struggling to cope with the demands being made, particularly in the light of demographic pressures from older people needing support to remain in their own homes, and from the increasing numbers of people with mental health problems housed in the community. The way forward, argued the Commission, would require changes at both local and national levels, in particular:

• Better understanding of the housing and support needs of local communities, and evaluation of how well current provision meets such needs.

• Making better use of resources available, including: clarifying the role of sheltered housing and ensuring it is fit for its current role; reducing delays in adapting properties; and ensuring personal support for vulnerable people is available by shifting from crisis response to early intervention.

- Developing more effective working relationships between agencies and departments.

- Promoting the use of performance measures and Best Value principles.

- Better policy co-ordination between lead government departments, and reform of the funding regime.[37]

Table 2.1 The contribution of housing authorities and registered social landlords to community care

Housing services provided	Beneficiaries
Community alarms	More than 1.1 million older people
Aids and adaptations	125,000 Disabled Facilities Grants made since 1991, plus an unknown but significant number of council house adaptations
Home improvement agencies	Nearly 200 agencies nationally provide assistance with repairs and grants
Vulnerable single homeless	45,000 people with mental health problems, 40,000 physically disabled and 45,000 older people have been accepted as homeless since 1990
Specialised housing	450,000 units of sheltered housing with on-site wardens for older people
	82,000 units of supported housing for people with mental health problems, physical disabilities, learning disabilities, and other needs
Mainstream housing with support	Housing agencies provide extra support to enable vulnerable people to maintain their tenancy, e.g. helping older people with gardening, or regular visits from housing officers. Provision of support is not consistently defined or recorded

Source: Audit Commission. *Home alone: the role of housing in community care*. London: Audit Commission, 1998, Exhibit 1

2.42 Shortly after the Audit Commission report was published, the Department of Social Security issued a consultation document, *Supporting People*.[38] In place of *ad hoc* funding through housing benefit, the paper proposed a simplified funding stream. This would introduce a specific grant for local authorities to provide a broad range of support services helping vulnerable people to live independently in the community. From 2003, the *Supporting People* programme will redirect funding towards services to help people live independently and to integrate support with wider local strategies. The funding is to be used to support housing-related services and to be complementary to existing care services. The aim is to provide housing support to vulnerable people and to improve the quality and effectiveness of supported housing in the following ways:

- more systematically focusing on local need
- breaking the link between support services and tenure
- promoting a wider range of services
- integrating support with wider local strategies
- monitoring and inspection according to Best Value
- transparent and cost-effective decision-making.[39]

2.43 The new model of funding set out in *Supporting People* gives local authorities the responsibility for making decisions on expenditure on local support services, so bringing together housing, social services and probation. It *does not* provide for people who need intensive levels of personal care. This should be provided through the route of community care assessments, although support is seen as complementary to existing care services. The new approach has been generally welcomed, as Fletcher has observed:

> *The aim is to achieve a more flexible person-centred funding system, though at the price of bringing in a cash limited control of expenditure, needs assessment for support services and prioritising between client groups. In terms of developing an integrated approach to funding support services for vulnerable people in regeneration areas and on a*

locality basis, the proposals nevertheless represent a major opportunity.[40]

2.44 However, the shift to a simplified funding stream represents a change away from a demand-led system based on individual rights through entitlement based on receipt of benefit. The new system of cash-limited funding and entitlement is based on assessment of need. The policy has been presented as a key component of the Government's strategy for promoting social inclusion. The approach is potentially more flexible than previous policies focusing on supported housing, particularly as people do not have to be resident in special housing schemes to receive support services. Under the *Supporting People* programme, for example, local authorities will be able to:

- help older people remain in their own homes by funding visiting support services

- continue to provide services in sheltered housing schemes

- help young people leaving care prepare for greater independence through training in basic skills such as cooking and hygiene

- help people leaving institutions, such as prison, or who have been homeless, with setting up home

- provide on-going support for people adjusting to more independent living.[41]

2.45 A review of the *Supporting People* programme carried out for the Joseph Rowntree Foundation concluded that there was evidence of 'genuine progress towards a more coherent approach to supporting independent living across Government departments, particularly in recognising the need for co-ordinated planning locally'.[42]

Regeneration

2.46 The regeneration agenda is closely linked to that of housing, and includes initiatives both within the DETR and the Social Exclusion Unit. Growing gaps between the richest and poorest in modern Britain have been highlighted by the Social Exclusion Unit. The poorest neighbourhoods are characterised by multiple deprivations related to the decline of traditional industries, the resulting high unemployment, and the difficulties of social and family fragmentation.[43]

2.47   Capital and revenue investment in areas of urban and rural poverty and deprivation have been features of government programmes for over 20 years. The approach has tended to focus on tightly defined geographic areas, and has been characterised by initiatives to improve living conditions within those areas. Since 1997, there has been a new emphasis on regeneration that has focused on neighbourhoods, involving the development of a range of partnership approaches. Funding from central government is managed through joint boards bringing together relevant local agencies. The Government's strategy for neighbourhood renewal has emphasised still more strongly the importance of having a neighbourhood focus for economic, social and physical regeneration. Local Area Strategic Partnerships are the means adopted to give this form, and to co-ordinate a range of different interventions.

2.48   There are four themes in the Government's approach to neighbourhood renewal:

- revival of the local economy
- engagement of the community in shaping and delivering local approaches
- full engagement of the independent sector
- developing and fostering local leadership.

These themes are of central importance to the debate about the provision of care and support. In particular, the development of the care sector is a key aspect of many local economies. The way in which this takes place will determine the nature of both the care provided and the employment created. Furthermore, the emphasis on local responses is critical.

2.49 Closely associated with the Neighbourhood Renewal Strategy, which is co-ordinated through the DETR, are a range of highly focused ('New Deal') initiatives designed to help specific groups of people enter, or re-enter, the labour market. These initiatives come under the umbrella of 'Welfare to Work'; they are targeted at specific groups of unemployed people, such as disabled people, and link training with entry to work. These initiatives are intended to respond to local labour market conditions.

2.50 A third relevant strand of economic regeneration are the powers local authorities have to engage with the local economy. Many authorities have used this to develop employment activities, sometimes by encouraging new small businesses and co-operatives. In the care and support sector, much of which is independent provision, the encouragement of small-scale businesses to meet identified gaps is an important part of economic regeneration.

Education and training

2.51 Education policy has, in many ways, been the distinguishing characteristic of the New Labour administration, with its central emphasis on raising educational standards in primary and secondary schools. Developments in training are particularly relevant to the focus of the Inquiry. As we explore later in Section 3 of the report, there is a fundamental need for more and better training in the care sector.

2.52 The 1999 education White Paper, *Learning to Succeed*,[44] set out its vision for a 'new culture of learning which will underpin national competitiveness and personal prosperity'. The framework for delivering this is built around three key objectives:

- to ensure that all young people reach 16 with the skills, attitudes and personal qualities that will give them a secure foundation for lifelong learning, work and citizenship in a rapidly changing world

- to develop in everyone a commitment to Lifelong Learning, to enhance their lives and improve their employability in a changing labour market, and to deliver the skills that the economy and employers need
- to help people without a job get into work.

2.53   The Learning and Skills Act (2000) established the National Learning and Skills Council, which will have responsibility for planning, funding, management, and quality assurance of all further education and training for those aged 16 years and over. Local Learning and Skills Councils will work with the National Training Organisations and the University for Industry to ensure that local training provision is well integrated with local skills needs. There are some 75 National Training Organisations (NTOs), covering more than 90 per cent of the workforce. Most focus on a particular industry, sector or service, with the two most relevant to the Inquiry known as TOPSS (the Training Organisation for the Personal Social Services) and Healthwork UK, the NTO for health. NTOs have a strategic role as the recognised voice of employers, and are particularly responsible for:

- identifying skill shortages and the training needs of the whole of their sector
- influencing and advising Government policy on education and careers guidance, and training arrangements and their solutions
- leading the development of qualifications based on national occupational standards, and advising on the national qualification structure.[45]

2.54   As has been noted previously, the importance of education and training has been recognised as part of the modernisation agenda in health and social care. The Department of Health's review of workforce planning, launched in September 1999, examined workforce planning issues for all professional groups within the NHS.[46] Workforce planning for the NHS was defined as ensuring sufficient staff are available with the right skills to deliver high-quality care to patients. Other work has also taken place in the development of a human resource strategy for nurses, professions allied to medicine (PAMs), scientists and technicians. Relatively little attention has been paid in such strategic documents to the contribution of many staff such as health care assistants. However, the NHS Plan has announced new investment to support a programme of training and development for *all* NHS staff. For professionally qualified staff, this has implications for continuing development and re-registration. For staff without a professional qualification:

> *Over the next three years we will guarantee all such staff access either to an Individual Learning Account of £150 a year or dedicated training to NVQ level two and three. This investment will help the NHS make better use of the potential of health care assistants, operating department practitioners, pharmacy technicians and others.*[47]

2.55   The NHS Plan gave welcome recognition to the long-standing neglect of the skills and potential of staff without professional qualifications. In signalling the need to make better use of the potential of health care assistants and other support staff, the Plan also acknowledged the need for effective regulation of these groups, and indicated that proposals would be forthcoming. A subsequent document on taking forward the NHS Plan re-stated the need to plan effectively for all NHS staff groups, and to end the historic division between planning for medical staff and for other health care professionals.[48] At a local level, all NHS organisations are to develop 'proper workforce plans'. From April 2001, 24 new Workforce Development Confederations will be established:

> *They will bring together NHS and non-NHS employers to plan the whole health care workforce, including medical staff, across wider communities, recognising that the NHS is not the only employer of health care staff.*[49]

2.56   These local confederations are to be paralleled by the reform of national planning arrangements and the establishment (also from April 2001) of a

National Workforce Development Board. The Board will in turn be supported by a number of care group workforce teams focusing on the workforce requirements for different care groups. These teams will cover the priority areas for which National Service Frameworks are also being developed, i.e. mental health, cancer services, coronary heart disease, children's services, and services for older people:

> *The teams will take a national view on the workforce development issues and challenges in their area, feeding into National Service Framework development and implementation, identifying workforce and education and training changes which may be needed as patterns of care change and making recommendations on staff requirements in their areas.*[50]

2.57   This brief overview has outlined some of the key developments in public policy and legislation that directly or indirectly shape the environment of health and care support workers. Underpinning all these developments, there are other factors, including shifting public expectations and the growing power of consumerism. Despite the considerable importance that has been given to 'joined-up government', it is apparent that many developments, apparently on on the periphery of the working environment, could have profound and largely uncontrolled (or unforeseen) consequences for employment in care and support. New European Directives in the employment field, for example, could have far reaching effects.

Demographic and social trends

2.58   The policy context is an important part of the environment shaping the provision and characteristics of care and support services. However, it does not exist in a vacuum and other important variables need also to be considered. Demographic and social trends affect both the demand and supply sides of the equation. That is, the likely need for care and support on the one hand, and the availability of an appropriate labour force on the other.

2.59   One starting point is the relative size of different cohorts of the total population. Although the total population of the UK continues to grow, the overall rate of growth is slowing. The main features of change include:

- the population is ageing, and fertility is falling
- the number of children aged under 16 is expected to fall by 9 per cent between 1996 and 2021
- the population of working age (defined by demographers as 16–64 years for men and 16–59 years for women) is expected to remain virtually static.

2.60   Table 2.2 presents key projections for the UK population over the next 30 years. The elderly, and very elderly, population is projected to continue to rise. In contrast, the number of people in those age groups from which support workers are usually drawn is expected to fall in both absolute and relative terms. Some key features can be identified:

- one person in six in the UK is aged at least 65; this will be true of one in four by 2031
- almost half the elderly population is aged at least 75
- the most rapid increases are projected to take place among those aged 85 years and over.

2.61   The growth and ageing of the population is characteristic of developed countries. The confluence of increasing life expectancy alongside falling fertility rates leads to an increase in the number *and proportion* of the older population.[51,52] The ageing of the population has often been described in negative terms, for example, as 'the demographic time bomb'. We do not subscribe to this alarmist interpretation, but we *do* recognise that the demands associated with the growth of the very elderly population are significant. Figure 2.3 graphically demonstrates the changing balance of the UK population by comparing the total numbers of people aged over 60 years with the numbers of younger adults aged in their 20s and 30s. In 2001, there were almost 40 per cent fewer people in the older age groups than in the younger adult groups. However, with the numbers in the younger group falling steadily, and those in the older groups rising, the proportions are shifting. By 2031, it is projected that the numbers of older people will outnumber the younger group by 24 per cent.

Table 2.2 Projected age structure of the UK population (1000s)

Age (years)	1996	2001	2011	2021	2031
0–14	11,358	11,288	10,508	10,369	10,276
	(19.3)	(18.9)	(17.2)	(16.7)	(16.4)
15–24	7,326	7,340	7,854	7,267	7,060
	(12.5)	(12.3)	(12.9)	(11.7)	(11.2)
25–34	9,420	8,461	7,541	8,054	7,476
	(16)	(14.2)	(12.4)	(12.9)	(11.9)
35–44	8,062	9,144	8,491	7,584	8,096
	(13.7)	(15.3)	(13.9)	(12.2)	(12.9)
45–54	7,596	7,851	9,016	8,378	7,501
	(13.0)	(13.2)	(14.8)	(13.5)	(11.9)
55–64	5,759	6,236	7,466	8,634	8,035
	(9.8)	(10.5)	(12.3)	(13.8)	(12.8)
65–74	5,058	4,893	5,451	6,596	7,738
	(8.6)	(8.2)	(8.9)	(10.6)	(12.3)
75–84	3,126	3,243	3,305	3,903	4,760
	(5.3)	(5.4)	(5.4)	(6.3)	(7.6)
85+	1,068	1,161	1,296	1,458	1,880
	(1.8)	(1.9)	(2.1)	(2.3)	(3.0)

Source: Office for National Statistics. *1996-based National Population Projections.* Government Actuary's Department. London: The Stationery Office, 1999

Figure 2.3: The changing age balance of the UK population

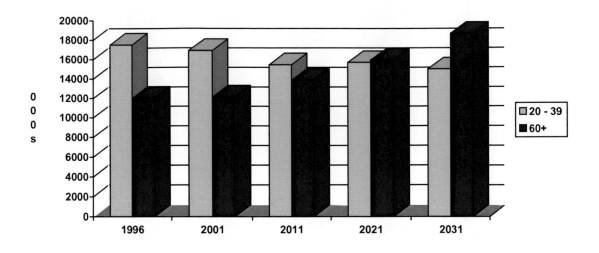

Older people from black and minority ethnic communities

2.62   The picture of the older population outlined above needs to be qualified by considering the variations that exist between different black and minority ethnic groups compared with the white population. In general terms, the minority ethnic population in Britain is younger than the white population, while there are also differences *between* various ethnic groups. The younger age profile of the black and minority ethnic communities primarily reflects the pattern of inward migration that occurred mainly in the 1950s and 1960s. The groups coming to Britain during that time came mainly as young adults and families, and provides the basis for the significant expansion of the older black and minority ethnic groups, which is increasingly evident. Between 1981 and 1991, it is estimated that the number of people of pensionable age in black and minority ethnic communities almost trebled (from 61,200 to 164,306).[1] The needs of future generations of black and minority ethnic older people will be of increasing significance, but will also change over time. For example, second-generation older people will be less likely to have the same level of English language and literacy needs as current older people. Table 2.3 summarises data taken from the last national census in 1991.

Table 2.3 Age structure of the black and minority ethnic population in Britain in 1991

Ethnic group	Structure of population (%) by age group					
	0–4 (%)	5–15 (%)	16–24 (%)	25–44 (%)	45–64 (%)	65+ (%)
White	6.5	13	12.9	29.3	19.2	19.3
Black	11.1	18	16.5	33.8	15.4	5.1
South Asian	10.9	24.6	16.5	30.5	13.5	3.9
Chinese and others	11.6	20.1	16.1	36.9	11.4	3.8

Source: Royal Commission on Long Term Care. *With Respect to Old Age, The Context of Long Term Care Policy, Research Volume 1.* Chapter 9: Black and Minority Ethnic Elderly: Perspectives on Long Term Care Table 1. London: The Stationery Office, 1999

2.63   Not only is the population profile of black and minority ethnic groups different from that of the white population, there are also important differences in health status. Despite the fact that black pensioners are comparatively younger overall than white pensioners, their health status is similar to that of older white pensioners. As other analyses have pointed out, greater levels of frailty and ill health should be seen in the context of poor economic and housing conditions, which are often the lifetime experience of these communities.[54] The concept of 'triple jeopardy' is sometimes applied to black and minority ethnic older people suffering cumulative disadvantage, in which racial discrimination compounds the disadvantages associated with old age, within a system of health and care support that inadequately recognises their needs. Triple jeopardy has been defined as the 'combined impact of race, age and social class on the lives of people in disadvantaged minorities'.[55] They are 'at risk because they are old, because of the physical conditions and hostility under which they have to live, and because services are not accessible to them'.[56]

2.64   The most extensive survey on the health of black and minority ethnic communities carried out to date indicates:

- Chinese men and women are less likely than the general population (by about 40 per cent), and less likely than all other minority groups, to report limiting long-standing illness.

- Pakistani and Bangladeshi men and women are three to four times more likely than the general population to rate their own health as bad or very bad. Indian men and women and black Caribbean women are also more likely to report poor health (although to a lesser extent).

- Bangladeshi and Pakistani men and women are more likely than the general population to score highly in a General Health Questionnaire, indicating that they are more likely to experience a psychiatric illness. Slightly higher scores were also found for black Caribbean and Indian women. By contrast, Chinese men and women are far *less* likely than the general population to have high scores.

- South Asian and Chinese men and women were at least twice as likely as the general population to be judged as having a severe lack of social support.[57]

- People from African Caribbean ethnic backgrounds are also over-represented in the diagnosis of psychoses. They are more likely to be referred to mental health services by the criminal justice system than by GPs or through social care routes.[58]

2.65   The National Service Framework for Older People also recognises that some illnesses are more prevalent among different minority groups, e.g. hypertension and stroke among African Caribbean people, and diabetes among South Asian individuals. As the National Service Framework emphasises, these differences will become increasingly significant as the population continues to age. The increased number of older people in black and minority ethnic communities underlines the importance of developing appropriate services. These will need to be accessible to all, with a culturally competent workforce, which reflects the diversity of local populations.

Health expectancy

2.66   The size of the older population is only a crude indicator of the likely needs for care or support, although there is a strong correlation between advancing years and increasing dependency. However, much depends on *health expectancy* as well as overall life expectancy. There is an ongoing debate over whether older people are living longer lives with *fewer* years of poor health, or whether they experience more ill health for longer. In reviewing the available evidence, the Royal Commission on Long Term Care concluded that there *is* an overall improvement in health expectancy. Although some 'compression of morbidity' *is* probably taking place, there is limited data to support this. The Commission was therefore cautious, and based its underlying assumptions on the premise that the proportion of years spent with disability will remain roughly the same in relation to overall life expectancy.[59]

2.67   The needs of the older population are changing, and conditions such as dementia and neurodegenerative diseases are becoming more significant. The incidence of dementia rises dramatically with age and doubles in each five-year age band over age 65. Thus, among people aged over 80, one in five are likely to be affected, compared to only one in 100 of those aged 65. Because of the growth of the oldest age groups, it is projected that the number of cases of dementia in the UK will double in the next 50 years to reach approximately two million.[60]

2.68   The Royal Commission also highlighted the limitations of data, which means that any projections about future needs are made with wide margins of uncertainty, and that there exists an expanding 'funnel of doubt' over likely scenarios. This doubt increases with time into the future. Although it gave projections up to 2051, the Commission emphasised that these were unlikely to be reliable beyond about twenty years. The recent emergence of conditions such as AIDS/HIV, and new variant Creutzfeldt-Jakob disease (CJD), are examples of how difficult it can be to predict the future.[61] There is considerable optimism in the scientific community, however, about the scope for preventing or reversing some chronic and degenerative conditions, not least through new techniques such as stem cell therapy and gene therapy. Nevertheless, while there *may* be enormous potential for such developments, it is also evident that this is an area of untried and uncertain science in which the rate of progress is uncertain and hoped-for outcomes may prove beyond reach. A vivid example of this is the treatment trials of Parkinson's disease using fetal cells implanted into the brains of patients with the condition. Initially promising results were followed a year after implant by an apparently irreversible worsening of symptoms.[62] Although other revolutionary interventions are likely to emerge, the needs of people with degenerative and chronic conditions are likely to be an increasing feature of the ageing population for the foreseeable future.

2.69   The Inquiry was not solely concerned with the care and support of older people. The needs of younger disabled people were also considered. The major source of information on disability is the now dated 1985 national survey.[63] The survey defined disability in terms of the lack of ability to perform normal activities resulting 'from the impairment of a structure or function of the body or mind'. The survey categorised disability in 10 bands of severity, and estimated that 6 million people in Britain have some sort of disability, with 70 per cent of these being aged over 60 years. Table 2.4 summarises some key data.

2.70   There are clear limitations to these data. The total numbers of disabled adults provides only a very broad indicator, and is of little sensitivity in discriminating between different types of disability. Those disabilities associated with mental incapacity or impairment may be overlooked, particularly with intermittent mental health problems. Table 2.5 summarises other estimates assembled by the Audit Commission from a range of sources.

Table 2.4 Estimated numbers of adults with a disability in Great Britain

Age group (years)	Number (1000s)	Rate per thousand
16–19	76	21
20–29	264	31
30–39	342	44
40–49	453	70
50–59	793	133
60–69	1,334	240
70–79	1,687	408
80+	1254	714
Total	**6,202**	**142**

Source: Martin J, Meltzer H, Elliot D. *OPCS surveys of disability in Great Britain 1985.* London: HMSO, 1988

Table 2.5 Estimated numbers of vulnerable people in the population

Client group	Estimated prevalence	Estimated number in England and Wales
Frail older people	1 in 40	1,300,000
Physical disability	1 in 100	500,000
Severe mental illness	1 in 250	200,000
Severe learning disabilities	1 in 250	200,000

Source: Audit Commission. *Home alone: the role of housing in community care.* London: Audit Commission, 1998, p.6, Table 1

2.71   Numbers alone give no indication of future trends. There are different factors likely to influence future developments in differing ways.

- Positive developments in neonatal care mean that more premature infants and babies born with complex needs now survive than was previously the case, but many of these will have physical or learning disabilities.

- Parallel developments in antenatal screening may reduce the numbers of children born with disabilities or special needs, either through interventions that can correct some conditions *in vitro*, or by terminations that prevent the birth of children with some conditions, such as Down's Syndrome.

- Developments in medical research will increasingly allow the treatment of disabling conditions for which there is currently no cure, e.g. research into stem cells and cloning may lead to new treatments for many chronic conditions.

2.72   Clearly, all these developments, and others, are likely to have profound consequences on the nature and prevalence of disability. They also raise major ethical and philosophical questions about the desirability or defensibility of interventions of this nature. Other relevant factors include:

- availability of informal care by family members, and to a lesser extent by friends and neighbours
- changing attitudes and expectations
- availability of a suitable labour force.

Informal care

2.73   The importance of informal care has been increasingly recognised in the last two decades, both in research and policy. It is estimated that there are 5.7 million people who provide some level of informal care. This means approximately 14 per cent of the adult population are carers.

2.74 As Table 2.6 demonstrates, the peak age for caring is between 45 and 64 years, with the largest group of carers being those who provide help to parents or parents-in-law. Carers looking after another household member are most likely to be caring for a spouse or partner.

Table 2.6 Percentage of adults who were carers, by age and sex

	Men			Women			Total		
Age group (years)	1985	1990	1995	1985	1990	1995	1985	1990	1995
16–29	6	7	5	7	9	6	7	8	6
30–44	11	12	8	16	18	13	14	15	10
45–64	16	20	17	24	27	22	20	24	20
65+	14	14	14	12	13	11	13	13	13
Total	**12**	**13**	**11**	**15**	**17**	**14**	**14**	**15**	**13**

Source: Office for National Statistics. *Informal Carers. Results of an independent study carried out on behalf of the Department of Health as part of the 1995 General Household Survey.* London: The Stationery Office, 1998, p.16, Table 4

2.75 Whether or not informal care will continue to be provided at current levels is a matter of great uncertainty. Any changes in the provision of informal care could have major implications for the consequent demands for formal care services. Policy in recent times has emphasised the need to support carers, epitomised in the publication in 1999 of the National Strategy for Carers. They have been praised as the 'unsung heroes of British life'.[64] However, there are many variables that *could* reduce the availability of carers in future years, including:

- changing patterns of family formation
- increased family breakdown
- smaller family size
- increased geographic mobility
- changing patterns of female employment
- shifting the balance between means-tested and 'free' care

- reduced willingness to take on caring roles.[65]

2.76 The impact of these trends can only be speculated on. For example, the Royal Commission on Long Term Care concluded that the likelihood of being married, and therefore having a spouse available as a potential carer, is in decline. However, the impact of other trends was much less clear, and for projection purposes, the Commission assumed that, other than allowing for the effects of a decline in marriage, there would be no real change in the future availability of informal care.

2.77 There is currently no evidence to indicate that people are less willing to care or to provide practical help to family members. However, we know relatively little about attitudes towards caring responsibilities and how these may have changed over time. The attitudes of people towards *receiving* help and support from family members are also important, and it is likely that these are changing. There is some evidence that people express a preference for professional rather than informal help so that they can maintain their dignity and autonomy.

2.78 A survey commissioned by Age Concern as part of the Millennium Debate of the Age asked people how they would prefer to be looked after if they could no longer manage to live independently. The findings (Table 2.7) indicated:

- a clear preference for remaining in their own home
- a greater preference for a mix of informal and professional support than for one or other alone
- informal care by relatives became less popular with advancing income.

Table 2.7 Preferences for formal and informal care

Imagine that some time in the future you could no longer manage on your own and needed help with daily tasks such as getting up, going to bed, feeding, washing or dressing, or going to the toilet. How would you like to be looked after?

Type of care	Gross personal income per annum				
	Less than £6,000	£6,000–£11,999	£12,000–£19,999	£20,000+	All
	(%)	(%)	(%)	(%)	(%)
Relatives in own home	19	16	13	8	15
Relatives in their home	4	3	1	–	3
Professionals in own home	19	21	19	25	21
Nursing or residential home	12	11	11	12	12
Mix of family and professionals in own home	42	45	55	53	47
Other	2	2	1	1	2
N (base)	667	459	299	285	1,710

Source: Jarvis C, Stuchbury R, Hancock R. *ACIOG Analysis of July 1997 ONS Omnibus Survey Data.* London: Age Concern Institute of Gerontology, King's College, 1998, Table A.6, p.19

2.79   In addition to specific attitudes and aspirations towards informal care, there is also a wider area of expectations that needs to be considered. Our expectations inevitably rise over time and yesterday's luxury soon becomes today's necessity. This has happened, for example, with consumer goods, but something similar probably also occurs in attitudes to services and support, whether in the public or private sector. In the note of dissent by Joffe and Lipsey to the report of the Royal Commission, it was argued that the

Commission's projections did not reflect adequately future expectations of quality, and that 'the demand for higher standards will be irresistible'. Such demands are likely to be evident in many forms. Joffe and Lipsey pointed, for example, to future demands for en suite bathroom facilities in care homes, and to the dissatisfaction of future generations with communal lounges and endless television as an answer to their recreational and leisure needs.[66] This is undoubtedly true, and successive cohorts of older people will have rising expectations for standards of care, particularly at a time of rising economic prosperity in society as a whole.

Economic and employment factors

2.80   The distinguishing feature of care and support is that it is essentially a 'high touch people industry'. This means it relies on the availability of people to provide personal, practical and emotional support to those in need of it. In future, some change might be expected. The development of new technologies, and the expansion of universal design principles, *could* result in a greater capacity of people to control their environments and to do things for themselves that would normally need other people's help. Examples include developments in assistive technology, particularly 'smart homes'. There are, however, clearly issues about the affordability of, and access to, such technology.[67,68] A Foresight report on the built environment and transport observed:

> *The growth of new technologies will present new and exciting challenges and opportunities for our sector. Digital technologies will enable us to interact more effectively with our physical environment, for example, through 'smart' housing and telematics in transport infrastructure. But, while technology may in many respects shrink the world we live in, the need and desire to travel and engage with others will remain as strong as ever.*[69]

2.81   Innovative approaches to a new generation of robots to provide 'companionship', as well as practical support to older people, are being developed in Japan and elsewhere. Whatever the scope of technology, there will continue to be a need for *people* to provide personal support and contact.

2.82   Changes in employment patterns over recent decades have been dramatic, and are characterised by the following trends:

- increased unemployment from the late 1970s to the mid-1990s
- the emergence of self-employment, short-term contracts and successive careers in place of the traditional pattern of 'a job for life'
- the expansion of women's economic activity (particularly in part-time employment)
- delayed entry into full-time employment, reflecting the parallel growth of further and higher education
- a trend towards 'early' retirement, particularly for males
- a decline in manufacturing employment and the rise of the service sector.[70]

2.83   A major problem with the service sector is the increasing under-supply of human resources. The Department of Health has acknowledged this difficulty in the NHS. In part, the problems are being tackled by more investment in developing human resources and expanding the number of places for people entering NHS training. The aim is to produce more doctors, nurses, therapists, etc., some years into the future. However, it is also recognised that this is only part of the solution, and the NHS Plan has indicated other approaches to the problem, including:

- modernising pay structures and increasing earnings
- improving the working lives of staff
- recruiting more staff from abroad.[71]

2.84   The 2001 Budget also announced various strategies to ease recruitment and retention difficulties both in the NHS and in the teaching profession, making use, in particular, of financial incentives and levers.

2.85   Similar difficulties exist in social care, but are not as yet being tackled by similar strategies. The 2000 annual report from the Chief Inspector of Social Services acknowledged that councils were reporting 'the utmost difficulty recruiting competent staff to fill posts which are critical to the delivery of the government's agenda'.[72] The solution to this problem is rather less clear, with the Chief Inspector saying only that:

> *Councils responsible for social care services also need to consider how they develop, recruit and retain essential staff. Councils are responsible for encouraging other employers to develop life long strategies; they should ensure that they too have such strategies for their own staff.*[73]

2.86   Alongside these 'domestic' factors, there are also wider considerations. The changing nature and structure of employment is influenced by developments elsewhere. Employment law is an area in which the influence of European Directives has been especially significant. While these Directives are typically concerned with improving the terms and conditions of employees, and safeguarding their health and safety, part of the price of this achievement may be a constraint on the flexibility of the labour force. Both the introduction of the National Minimum Wage and the EU Working Time Directive have contributed to pressures, particularly for small-scale service providers, who risk being squeezed out of the market.[74]

2.87   The 1998 White Paper, *Fairness at Work*, presented proposals for a series of measures, subsequently enacted in the Employment Relations Act (1999). A major focus of these proposals was improving the balance between work and home life. Accordingly, the Parental Leave Directive allows rights to parental leave, time off for family emergencies, and improved maternity rights. The Working Time Directive limits workers to a maximum of 48-hours work per week (unless they choose to work for longer). It introduces requirements for rest periods, time off, and annual leave, etc. Part-time workers are also protected against less favourable treatment through new regulations setting minimum standards for fair pay, pensions, training, and holiday entitlement. The Labour government also introduced a National Minimum Wage for adult employees (£3.70 an hour since October 2000 and £4.10 from April 2001); supervision of the minimum rate is the responsibility of the Low Pay Commission.

2.88   A further vital component of the labour force in the area of care and support is provided by what is termed 'the third sector', i.e. the voluntary sector. The voluntary, or non-profit sector, is a major employer. In 1995, the broad non-profit sector employed around 1.5 million full-time equivalent paid workers. If only the 'narrow voluntary sector' is counted, i.e. excluding organisations not traditionally part of the UK voluntary sector, there are still half a million employees, equivalent to half the size of the NHS workforce.[75,76] As Kendall and Almond point out, while the sector's contribution to paid employment is considerable, 'volunteering remains the primary labour input for the sector as a whole', with 16 million volunteers overall contributing the work of 1.7 million full-time equivalent employees.[77]

2.89   The expansion of volunteering is increasingly featured as an objective on the political agenda. The contribution of older people as volunteers was one of the themes of the BGOP programme and responding to the recommendations the Government endorsed older volunteers as 'a vital national resource'.[78] Further expansion of such activity is being encouraged through a 'National Experience Corps' aimed at involving volunteers aged over 50 years. This development may be attractive to government not only for the potential in mobilising extra human resources, but doing so in ways that promote broader political objectives of active citizenship and social inclusion. The Chancellor of the Exchequer, Gordon Brown, has similarly encouraged the giving both of money and time to voluntary action through a new 'civic patriotism', with the goal that within five years every citizen should be committed to giving two hours a week to the community. An extra £300 million is to be invested in developing community volunteering.[79] We return later in this report to consider the likely prospects for volunteering contributing to the development of care and support.

2.90   The purpose of this background section of the paper has been to outline the context for the Inquiry. It has included a wide range of factors and sketched a sweeping landscape. This is essential for understanding the issues which confront the care and support sectors. As Figure 2.1 at the beginning of this section demonstrates, the external environment is one of multiple influences. Some of these have a more direct relationship with health and care issues than others, but all are relevant. Unless they can all be taken into account, the capacity to influence change in care and support is extremely limited.

References

[1] Department of Health. *A quality strategy for social care.* London: Department of Health, 2000, para. 2.

[2] *Ibid.*

[3] Sutherland S. (Chairman) *With respect to old age: long term care – rights and responsibilities: A report by the Royal Commission on Long Term Care.* Cm 4192-I. London: The Stationery Office, 1999.

[4] *Ibid.*, p.10, Table 2.2.

[5] Griffiths R. *Community care: agenda for action. A report to the Secretary of State for Social Services.* London: HMSO, 1988.

[6] Secretaries of State. *Caring for people: community care in the next decade and beyond.* Cm 849. London: The Stationery Office, 1989.

[7] Central Policy Review Staff. *A joint framework for social policies.* London: HMSO, 1975.

[8] Secretary of State for Social Security. *Opportunity for all: tackling poverty and social exclusion. First annual report 1999.* Cm 4445. London: The Stationery Office, 1999.

[9] Macpherson, Sir William. *The Stephen Lawrence Inquiry. Report of an Inquiry by Sir William Macpherson of Cluny.* Cm 4262-I. London: The Stationery Office, 1999.

[10] Department of Health. *Human Rights Act 1998: European Convention on Human Rights case studies in health and social care.* London: Department of Health, 2000.

[11] Daw R. *Human rights and disability: the impact of the Human Rights Act on disabled people.* London: National Disability Council and Royal National Institute for the Deaf, 2000.

[12] Better Government for Older People. *All our futures: the report of the Better Government for Older People Steering Group.* Wolverhampton: Better Government for Older People, 2000.

[13] Inter-Ministerial Group for Older People. *Building on partnership: the government response to the recommendations of the Better Government for Older People programme.* London: Department of Social Security, 2000.

[14] Secretaries of State, 1989. *Op. Cit.*

[15] Secretary of State for Health. *Modernising social services: promoting independence, improving protection, raising standards.* Cm 4169. London: The Stationery Office, 1998.

[16] *Ibid.*, para. 1.7.

[17] Department of Health. *New 'concordat' proposed for care home sector. Extra £105 million to improve disability equipment services in the NHS.* Press release no. 2000/0705. 30 November, 2000.

[18] Hudson B. Modernising social services – a blueprint for the new millennium? In: Hudson B, editor. *The changing role of social care.* Research Highlights in Social Work 37. London: Jessica Kingsley, 2000.

[19] Knapp M, Hardy B, Forder J. Commissioning for quality: ten years of social care markets in England. *Journal of Social Policy* 2001; 27: 2.

[20] Milburn A. Keynote speech. Social Services Conference, Torquay. 29 October, 2001.

[21] Secretary of State for Health. *The NHS plan: a plan for investment; a plan for reform.* Cm 4818–I. London: The Stationery Office, 2000.

[22] *Ibid.*, para. 7.3.

[23] *Ibid.*, para. 7.4.

[24] Department of Health. *Intermediate care 2001.* HSC 2001/01. LAC (2001)1. 19 January.

[25] Secretary of State for Health, 2000. *Op. Cit.*, para. 7.10.

[26] Neate P. Hutton sets the pace but can the workers keep up? *Community Care* 2000; November 9–15: 10–11.

[27] Secretary of State for Health, 2000. *Op. Cit.*, para. 1.1.

[28] Hudson B. 2000, *Op. Cit.*, p. 224.

[29] *Ibid.*, p. 224

[30] Department of Health. *Modern standards and service models: mental health National Service Framework.* London: Department of Health, 1999.

[31] Department of Health. *Modern standards and service models: older people National Service Framework.* London: Department of Health, 2001.

[32] Department of Health. *A quality strategy for social care.* London: Department of Health, 2000, para. 29.

[33] Department of Health, 2000. *Op. Cit.*, para. 21.

[34] Secretary of State for Health. *The new NHS: modern, dependable.* Cm 3807. London: The Stationery Office, 1997.

[35] Department of the Environment/Department of Health. *Housing and community care.* London: DoE/DoH, 1992.

[36] Audit Commission. *Home alone: the role of housing in community care.* London: The Audit Commission, 1998.

[37] *Ibid.* Recommendations, pp 82–85.

[38] Department of Social Security. *Supporting people: a new policy and funding framework for support services.* London: Department of Social Security, 1998.

[39] Department of the Environment, Transport and the Regions (DETR). *Supporting people: together towards 2003.* London: DETR, 2000.

[40] Fletcher P. *Social inclusion for vulnerable people: linking regeneration and community care – the housing, care and support dimensions.* Brighton: Pavilion Publishing, 2000.

[41] Department of the Environment, Transport and the Regions (DETR). *Together towards 2003.* Supporting People Newsletter, 2000. (www.supporting.people.detr.gov.UK/news/tt2003/index.htm)

[42] Griffiths S. *Findings: an overview of the supporting people programme.* York: Joseph Rowntree Foundation, 2000.

[43] Social Exclusion Unit. *Bringing Britain together: national strategy for neighbourhood renewal.* London: The Cabinet Office, 2000.

[44] Department for Education and Employment. *Learning to succeed.* London: Department for Education and Employment, 1999.

[45] Department for Education and Employment, National Training Organisations, Web site information.

[46] Department of Health. *A health service of all the talents: developing the NHS workforce. Consultation document on the review of workforce planning.* London: Department of Health, 2000.

[47] Secretary of State for Health, 2000. *Op. Cit.*, para. 9.13.

[48] Department of Health. *Investment and reform for NHS staff – taking forward the NHS Plan.* London: Department of Health, 2001, para. 5.5

[49] *Ibid.*, para. 5.5.

[50] *Ibid*, para. 5.9.

[51] Henwood M. *The future of health and care of older people: the best is yet to come. The millennium papers.* Age Concern Debate of the Age. London: Age Concern England, 1999.

[52] Sutherland S, 1999. *Op. Cit.*, pp. 13–15.

[53] Department of Health, 2001. *Older people National Service Framework. Op. Cit.*, p. 3.

[54] Butt J, Mirza K. *Social care and black communities.* London: HMSO, 1996.

[55] Blakemore K, Boneham M. *Age, race and ethnicity: a comparative approach.* Buckingham: Open University Press, 1994: p. 40.

[56] Norman A. *Triple jeopardy: growing old in a second homeland.* London: Centre for Policy on Ageing, 1985: p. 1.

[57] Joint Health Survey Unit. *Health survey for England: The health of minority ethnic groups '99. Summary of key findings.* London: Joint Health Surveys Unit, National Centre for Social Research, Department of Epidemiology and Public Health at the Royal Free and University College Medical School, 2001.

[58] *Ibid.*, Chapter 2, pp. 4–13.

[59] *Ibid.*, Chapter 2, p. 20.

[60] Khaw K-T. How many, how old, how soon? *BMJ* 1999; 319: 1350–2.

[61] Office for National Statistics. *1996-based national population projections. Prepared by the Government Actuary in consultation with the Registrars General.* Series PP2 No. 21. London: The Stationery Office, 1999.

[62] Boseley S. Parkinson's miracle cure turns into a catastrophe. *The Guardian* 2001, 13 March: 1.

[63] Martin J, Meltzer H, Elliot D. *OPCS surveys of disability in Great Britain 1985.* London: HMSO, 1988.

[64] Blair T. Foreword. In: *Caring about carers: a national strategy for carers.* London: The Stationery Office, 1999.

[65] Henwood M, 1999. *Op. Cit.*

[66] Joffe J, Lispey D. 'Note of Dissent'. In: Sutherland S, 1999. *Op. Cit.*

[67] *Findings: the market potential for smart homes.* York: Joseph Rowntree Foundation, 2000.

[68] Cowan D, Turner-Smith A. The role of assistive technology in alternatives models of care for older people. Appendix 4. Research Volume 2. In: *With respect to old age.* Cm 4192-I. London: The Stationery Office, 1999.

[69] Foresight. *The physical world in a virtual age.* Built Environment and Transport Panel. London: Department of Trade and Industry, 2000.

[70] Scales J, Pahl R. *Future work and lifestyles, the millennium paper.* Age Concern Debate of the Age. London: Age Concern England, 1999.

[71] Secretary of State for Health, 2000. *Op. Cit.*, Chapter 5. Investing in NHS staff: p. 51

[72] Social Services Inspectorate. *Modern social services: a commitment to people. The ninth annual report of the Chief Inspector of Social Services 1999/2000.* London: Department of Health, 2000.

[73] *Ibid.*, para. 1.20.

[74] Knapp M, Hardy B, Forder J, 2001. *Op. Cit.*, p. 2.

[75] Kendall J, Almond S. *The UK voluntary (third) sector in comparative perspective: exceptional growth and transformation.* London: PSSRU, London School of Economics. PSSRU, LSE; Charities Aid Foundation; Joseph Rowntree Foundation; The John Hopkins Comparative Non-profit Sector Project, 1998.

[76] Almond S, Kendall J. *Paid employment in the self-defined voluntary sector in the late 1990s: an initial description of patterns and trends.* Civil Society Working Paper No. 7. London: Centre for Civil Society, London School of Economics, 2000.

[77] Kendall J, Almond S, 1998. *Op. Cit.*, p. 2.

[78] Inter-Ministerial Group on Older People, 2001. *Op. Cit.*, p. 21.

[79] Speech by Gordon Brown to National Council of Voluntary Organisations (NCVO) annual conference. February 9, 2000.

3   Findings and analysis

3.1   The previous section set out the background to the Inquiry and highlighted the environment that both directly and indirectly shapes the world of care and support. An understanding of that environment, and of its complex interconnections, is fundamental to any discussion of the future of care and support and of raising the quality of services. We have emphasised that it is not sufficient to focus simply on the immediate policy developments in health and social care. Wider developments in the economy, the labour market, in European Directives and legislation and in socio-demographic trends can all have a significant effect on the way in which care and support services are organised and operate.

3.2   In this section, we consider the issues and themes identified in the course of the Inquiry. As we outlined at the beginning of this report, the Inquiry has focused on the quality of physical, practical and emotional support to adults in need of help because of frailty in old age, mental health problems, physical disability, chronic illness, or learning disability. In exploring the key dimensions of problems in care and support, our analysis was informed by rich and varied evidence. The King's Fund Commission members brought their own wealth of knowledge and experience. Alongside this, we were able to draw on a large volume of written submissions and from detailed discussions with an extensive range of individuals and organisations (see Appendix 2).

3.3   A vast range of issues were identified. However, several key themes were apparent, which formed the analytical framework for the Inquiry's findings:

- cost and quality
- skills and values of staff
- employment
- regulation and training
- management.

Cost and quality

3.4   A central theme running throughout our analysis was the tension arising from trying to achieve an acceptable service quality while containing overall costs. Raising the quality of services is at the heart of the Government's strategy for social care. John Hutton MP, Minister of State for Health, has underlined the radical change required to deliver services that are:

- able to respond to rising public expectations

- more accessible, consistent and convenient

- able to ensure the safety and protection of vulnerable children and adults

- able to promote independence.[1]

> *To rise to this challenge we need a new vision and culture in social services. Social services have serious responsibilities in law, and a duty to carry these out to the highest possible standards. We need to redesign radically our approach to delivery, planning and managing social services, by improving protection and extending choice, control and flexibility to those who need these vital services.*[2]

3.5   We would certainly endorse this vision, but the Inquiry found a large gulf between these aspirations and many people's routine experiences of using services. Shortcomings are extensive and include:

- use of unskilled and untrained care and support staff; and accompanying risks of injury and abuse

- poor responsiveness to the needs and wishes of service users

- insufficient sensitivity to the needs and preferences of black and minority ethnic groups

- lack of focus on enabling service users to lead independent lives, and a preoccupation with 'looking after' people

- inadequately developed models of service in which objectives are unclear and outcomes rarely identified.

As discussed later in this section, there are additional concerns about the employment conditions of staff in care and support services, especially:

- poorly paid employment which exploits the good will and commitment of staff

- services which afford inadequate protection, respect or dignity to individual support workers.

Users' views on quality

3.6   Evidence to support these findings comes from a variety of sources. There is an increasing amount of qualitative research literature exploring service users' experiences and perceptions. This literature is notable for the consistency of messages arising, and many of these themes were also underlined in our consultations with service users. It is apparent that service users' definitions of 'quality' focus not only on the material aspects of quality (such as the characteristics of a residential facility), but on the nature of the relationship with members of staff and the quality of their interaction with service users. A consultation by the National User Group, 'Shaping Our Lives', carried out to inform the development of codes of conduct and practice in social care, concluded the following:

> *The phrase 'putting the person first' emerged in the course of the meetings as a way of summing up virtually all of the comments about the positive ways services treat users and how users want to be treated in relation to the proposed codes of conduct and practice. Failure to put the person first also summed up many of the negative experiences and the conduct and practice that users would like to be deemed unacceptable by the codes.*[3]

3.7   Work with older people using domiciliary services carried out by the Nuffield Institute similarly found:

... that the satisfaction or dissatisfaction of clients receiving home care is primarily a reflection of the nature of their relationship with the home care staff on the one hand, and of the manner in which care is delivered on the other.[4]

The Nuffield Institute research found that service users defined a quality home care service as one characterised by the following features:

- staff reliability
- continuity of care and of staff
- kindness and understanding of care workers
- cheerfulness and demeanour of care staff
- competence in undertaking specific tasks
- flexibility to respond to changing needs and requirements
- knowledge and experience of the needs and wishes of the service user.

3.8 Similarly, work by the National Institute for Social Work with different groups of service users has identified the dimensions of quality of relationships, quality of skills and quality of services, and concluded:

It is easy to summarise what people who use services and carers value in their contacts with social services workers: they value courtesy and respect, being treated as equals, as individuals, and as people who make their own decisions; they value workers who are experienced, well informed and reliable, able to explain things clearly and without condescension, and who 'really listen'; and they value workers who are able to act effectively and make practical things happen.[5]

3.9 Submissions to the Inquiry reinforced these messages, including consultations with service users about the quality of the relationship with care staff (see Appendix 2). Box 3.1 summarises some of the key issues identified by service users during consultation. The issues reflect a wide range of concerns, and we will return to many of the themes.

3.10   It is perhaps easy to see concerns about the relationship between service users and support staff as relatively minor matters. However, we would argue that they are fundamentally important, not least because they are indicative of many other actual or potential problems, including:

- failure to treat service users as people first can lead to dehumanising treatment and actual abuse

- shortcomings point to wider problems with recruitment of appropriate care staff

- vital aspects of service quality are undermined by cost pressures which limit the capacity of services to respond.

Box 3.1 Views of service users from consultation meetings with the Inquiry

- Lack of understanding and compassion on the part of care workers.
- Lack of understanding of empowerment or enabling independence; care workers concerned instead with 'looking after'.
- In both subtle and overt ways, service users are often bullied by care and support staff.
- Lack of staff time and lack of appropriate skills.
- Services do not provide what people really need or want.
- Problems of continuity of care, particularly with high staff turnover.
- Institutionalised discrimination against older people in services, with lower cost ceilings for services than for younger people.
- Charging policies are a major deterrent for people who really need services.
- Direct Payments can offer a way forward, but are not appropriate for everyone.
- It is very difficult to make complaints. There is a fear of the consequences of 'whistle blowing', and an unwillingness to get staff into trouble.
- Lack of attention to needs of black and minority ethnic groups.
- Fears over future of social care and the risks of it being taken over by the NHS, which is seen as 10–15 years behind in its attitudes to disability.
- Particular problems at transition from children's to adult services, and from younger adults to elderly.
- How do you ensure a quality service when the prime motive of providers is that of profit?
- Workers cannot empower service users unless they themselves are empowered.
- Important aspects of support are not seen as core parts of the job and do not get done (particularly in interacting with people and encouraging communication and engagement).
- Care staff have become too professionalised to get involved in individual interaction.

Source: Views of service users from consultation meetings undertaken by the Inquiry

---

3.11   Another aspect of service quality is the poor access to services for specific groups of people. The 1998 social services White Paper, *Modernising Social Services*, highlighted recent research findings on the poor responsiveness of services, in terms of 'language barriers, assessment procedures and services which do not recognise cultural differences, and an over-reliance on the willingness and capacity of black families and carers to look after each other'.[6] There is evidence that black and minority ethnic groups are significantly disadvantaged as users of public services, as the Commission for Racial Equality has argued:

> *Ethnic minorities are both under- and over-represented as users of health and social care services. Typically, where care is more akin to control and brings restrictions on users' autonomy, ethnic minorities are over-represented. Where the services are 'caring', ethnic minorities tend to be under-represented. This is particularly apparent in mental health services.*[7]

3.12   Research commissioned by the Royal Commission on Long Term Care explored the perspectives of black and minority ethnic elderly people, and confirmed the inadequacy of mainstream providers 'and the compensatory effect of minority ethnic organisations who continue to act as 'primary providers'.[8] This was viewed as *de facto* racism with mainstream services structuring the segmentation of care by default, so that services for black and minority ethnic groups tended to be 'inadequately supported, maintained nor expanded'. Service users, and potential users from black and minority ethnic groups, often face problems of limited choice, poor information, cultural and language barriers and underlying discrimination.

3.13   Inadequate mainstream support for black and minority ethnic groups lies both in a lack of supply (poor range and choice of services), and in culturally inappropriate services. The Department of Health inspection of community care services for black and minority ethnic older people identified successful policies and strategies that had 'faced the issues of race and incorporated these into the mainstream of their considerations'.[9] The picture *is* one of some improvement, though also one of considerable variability between local authorities. Local ethnic minority groups and agencies have often been successful in developing innovative and successful services. However, as the Department of Health report notes, the majority of these groups are small in size, and they have little organisational infrastructure or experience of the contractual culture, a possible, significant disadvantage in competing as service providers.

3.14　The report of the Macpherson Inquiry into the death of Stephen Lawrence and its handling by the Metropolitan Police provides a framework both for identifying and tackling 'institutional racism' throughout public services. Institutional racism has been defined as:

> *... the collective failure of an organisation to provide appropriate and professional service to people because of their colour, culture and ethnic origin. It can be detected in processes, attitudes and behaviour which amount to discrimination through unwitting prejudice, ignorance, thoughtlessness and racist stereotyping which disadvantage minority ethnic people.*[10]

There is a major equalities agenda in care and support services which needs to be addressed both in the development of high-quality services and in establishing employment opportunities. We return to the latter in a subsequent section of the report.

3.15　Other submissions to the Inquiry have emphasised the 'double jeopardy' of race issues. The Sainsbury Centre for Mental Health has highlighted the over-representation of black service users in mental health services, particularly at the upper end of the Care Programme Approach (the CPA provides a framework for assessing the needs of, and planning services for, people accepted into specialist mental health services. It operates on a number of levels depending on the severity of the needs identified). They speculate that racist stereotypes may play a part, in which black service users are more likely to be identified as high risk than white users in terms of presenting a danger to others:

> *Black users are more likely to find themselves on the top tier of the CPA [Care Approach Programme] to begin with and, once there, the quality of their experience will be different not least because they are identified as risky.*[11]

3.16   Boxes 3.2 and 3.3 outline two positive examples of services developed to meet the needs of black and minority ethnic service users that were drawn to the attention of the Inquiry. Examples of innovative and responsive services in this area appear often to have originated from black and minority ethnic-led voluntary organisations in a 'bottom-up' approach. There *are* examples of good providers elsewhere, including some responsive and flexible local authority services. However, we need to address why pockets of good practice have tended to remain isolated and are slow to be incorporated into the mainstream. There are probably many relevant factors, including pressures from existing and potential service users, action from front-line staff and their managers, and effective advocacy by black and minority ethnic voluntary organisations.[12] Encouraging the spread of innovative developments on the ground is critical, particularly if they are to become mainstream rather than 'specialist' and often marginal. The qualities of good specialist services identified by service users are typically those associated with the skills and knowledge of staff, and with the respectful and non-stereotypical way in which services are delivered, rather than qualities associated with black workers *per se*. These factors are very similar to those generally identified by service users as contributing to quality services. Thus, the challenge is not just about developing a range of different services to meet the needs of black and minority ethnic groups, but also, more demandingly, that appropriate skills, knowledge and attitudes are developed in *all* workers.

Enabling people to take control

3.17 'Empowerment' is an issue that is identified frequently by service users. It refers to a change in power relationships whereby the focus of services is to assist the individual to achieve his or her goals. Enabling a person to achieve independence has implications for the type of support provided, as well as for the manner in which it is delivered. Many service users' experiences of services are quite different from such a model, and accounts of patronising and oppressive services that do not deliver what is wanted are frequently encountered. A lack of choice over how and when services are delivered, and having to fit in with service routines, rather than having services that respond to individual needs, are illustrative of the lack of power identified frequently in the research literature, and repeated in our investigation.

3.18 Some service users are less likely to have even a modicum of control and choice. The situation of younger adults with learning disabilities, or with mental health problems, who remain living in the parental home, for example, was highlighted in submissions to the Inquiry as one of little opportunity for independence. Similarly, the situation of people living in residential settings, rather than in the community, is often one of diminished control and little chance for autonomy.

3.19 The contrast between the type of support service that is generally available and that which service users would actually prefer can be identified. This is evident both in the private purchasing of services, and in the use of Direct Payments. The privately purchased care market has expanded along with the growth of the independent sector providing care and support services commissioned by local authorities. According to the Audit Commission's report on charging for home care services, authorities tend to impose cost ceilings on the amount of service they will provide to a user (often related to the costs of a residential placement):

> *Therefore, users with relatively high levels of need might be faced with a need to buy in large amounts of care over and above that provided by*

the council if they wish to stay in their own home. Related to this has been a general tightening of eligibility criteria, so those clients with lower levels of dependency are now less likely to receive services.[13]

Box 3.2 Innovative and added value services for black and minority ethnic groups: *'Mushkil Aasaan': supporting the community*

An innovative example of a domiciliary service supporting the black and minority ethnic community is that of Mushkil Aasaan, an approved provider in Wandsworth. As its publicity leaflet states, Mushkil Aasaan was established by a group of women *'who shared concerns about the plight of families experiencing crisis, social isolation and a complexity of unmet needs with little or no support networks. It now provides a generic model of support to families and elderly in need'.*

Discontent with services failing to provide culturally appropriate care led to the setting up of the service. A strong ethos of caring about each other and a commitment to meeting the needs of a diversity of clients. The strengths of the model include:

- Capacity to provide additional support, e.g. advocacy, is facilitated through the use of volunteers backing-up paid care staff.
- Recruitment of staff relies heavily on word of mouth within the community and is successful in attracting people who would often not be economically active.
- The provision of a culturally appropriate and sensitive service is highly valued both by service users and care staff.
- Serving the community is a prime motivation, which contributes to the status of the work and the expressed satisfaction of care workers.
- Care staff receive considerable support and back-up through their managers, and are given additional help with literacy and language skills.

Box 3.3 Innovative and added value services for black and minority ethnic groups: *Tooting Neighbourhood Centre: no boundaries to caring*

Tooting Neighbourhood Centre (TNC) is a long-established community organisation in South London, which since 1996 has had approved provider status to provide home care and respite. As with Mushkil Aasaan, TNC started out to meet a gap in the home care market and the inappropriateness or insensitivity of mainstream services to meet the needs of black older people. Although TNC started out to provide support to black older people who were not accessing the support they required, the service has been extended and almost half of the service users are white.

Strengths of the TNC service include:

- Users have direct contact with a local community organisation rather than a faceless agency, and the duty manager contacts all clients considered vulnerable by 'phone each evening to check they are all right.
- Care staff often undertake services beyond their specified duties (such as giving help with form filling, making appointments, etc.).
- Service users have access to a wide range of TNC's grant-aided and voluntary services and activities, such as luncheon club, day trips, counselling and befriending.

3.20 As the Commission observes, charges can affect users' decisions to use other care providers. Indeed, some councils have set charges for better-off service users at a level where it is more economical for them to obtain services directly from private providers:

> *Where council charges are close to or above the charges of private providers, users may have a strong incentive to use private provision instead – particularly as private providers can be more flexible.*[14]

3.21 The United Kingdom Home Care Association (UKHCA) similarly points to 'anecdotal evidence from providers', whereby people pay home care providers directly for additional care above the ceiling imposed by their social services departments, or pay for additional time 'in order for workers to undertake jobs considered inessential by care managers'.[15]

3.22   Direct Payments are seen by some as a useful way forward in changing the balance of power and placing control in the hands (and wallet) of the service user. For certain service users, Direct Payments enable people who have had a community care assessment to receive a regular cash payment instead of services to meet their assessed needs. Direct Payments are typically used to employ personal assistants 'to provide the support and help they need, at the times and in the manner determined by the disabled employer'.[16] The significance of Direct Payments lies not only in the scope for improving the responsiveness of services, but also in what the service provides. As pointed out by Glendinning *et al.*, the concept of independent living:

> *... embraces the twin principles of **choice** – over where and how to live and who provides assistance; and **control** – over when, where and how that assistance is provided. Independent living emphasises the ability to determine and fulfil chosen goals and lifestyles, with whatever assistance is needed in order to do so.*[17]

3.23   It is these dimensions of choice and control that are often notably absent from the organisation and delivery of support services, whereby critical decisions and choices are made on behalf of service users by others. The benefits for some of using Direct Payments are clear:

> *With personal assistants, both the timing of the help which users received and the manner in which this help was given could be tailored to their personal preferences and lifestyles. Their personal assistance was no longer fragmented between a number of different professionals, who might come at times which were inconvenient to users. Instead, direct payment users were able to choose who provided help with the different elements of their personal assistance needs; they were able to*

train their personal assistants to provide this help in ways which best suited them; and they felt less dependent on the good will of family and close friends.[18]

3.24   Other qualitative research on the use of payments, by Zarb and Nadash, has similarly emphasised the central importance of choice and control, for example:

> *I am in control. I can decide when I want help. The way help is delivered – I feel it is my life, not someone else's. You are not fitted in to other people's time table. Freedom – you can choose who you have. If you don't like them you can have someone else. You can choose the manner in which a task is performed, unlike when home care staff are used. It releases me to have family as family and friends as friends.*[19]

3.25   Clearly, as Zarb and Nadash argue, 'control' is multifaceted. It includes control over the type of assistance provided, how and when it is provided, and by whom. Wider benefits also arise in terms of enhanced personal freedom, relationships with others, and general quality of life.[20]

3.26   However, Direct Payments are never going to be appropriate for all service users (though arguably they should be an option for everyone), and many people find the idea of managing their own services daunting. Ways need to be found to incorporate the valued features of the direct payment model into the organisation of mainstream care and support.

3.27   Moreover, Direct Payments do not offer a panacea to all the problems involved in providing high-quality care. There are also some indications that employees may be disadvantaged in working as personal assistants. Analysis of this area undertaken by Glendinning *et al.* has emphasised, for example, how personal assistants are less likely than other care workers to have clearly defined roles or job descriptions. They may also experience problems in negotiating their role:

... [none of the] personal assistants [were] aware of any guidelines as to what they could or could not be expected to do; the tasks they carried out were negotiated on an individual basis between employer and employee. Some personal assistants reported considerable difficulty in conducting these negotiations and establishing boundaries around the range of activities they were expected to carry out.[21]

3.28   Personal assistants can also be vulnerable because of inadequate training for the tasks they undertake. Although their employer trains them for the work they do, some personal assistants feel they are carrying out tasks that they are not properly trained to do. This is particularly likely with specific health care tasks:

Those assistants who had received some instruction from health professionals ... reported that this had nevertheless been severely limited. Any such training often took the form of simply watching a particular procedure being performed by a health professional, perhaps on only one occasion, with no subsequent check to ensure that the quality of care was being sustained.[22]

3.29   The personal assistants voiced concerns about possible risks both to themselves, such as from infection, and to their employer, such as risk of injury. Some were also concerned over the general implications of carrying out tasks in the health domain with inadequate skills and training, especially issues of accountability and liability. Health and Safety rules governing the lifting or moving of service users were often identified by service users as being impractical and a source of problems. For example, a rule that prevents a paid member of staff from moving someone without help is intended for the protection of the employee, but can lead to service users not being able to move when they want to, or having to rely on family carers who are then themselves at risk of injury. Service users, particularly those who use personal assistants, have argued that there are safe, moving techniques capable of protecting both the service user and the employee. Indeed, a survey undertaken by the National Centre for Independent Living found that, of 124 personal assistants working for disabled individuals over a three-year period, *none had sustained any back injury while at work.*[23] Adequate training and skills are therefore of obvious importance, and we return to consider such issues more fully at a later stage.

3.30   The interests of personal assistants as employees are clearly important, and there may be some tensions that need to be addressed. However, the value of the greater control that service users experience in being able to employ workers directly, and to make choices about the type of person they want, are of central importance. When service users are the employers of personal assistants, they have considerable power, including that of 'hire and fire', and specification of the tasks to be undertaken. It is also recognised that this entails certain responsibilities and demands. Nonetheless, as Zarb and Nadash conclude, 'most people clearly feel that the responsibilities and effort involved with managing their own support arrangements are outweighed by the advantages'.[24]

Empowerment and user involvement

3.31   A frequent response to issues of empowerment is to call for 'greater user involvement', but what does this mean in practice? Clearly, there are both individual and collective dimensions. In terms of the latter, a positive way forward may lie in the greater involvement of service users in monitoring and reviewing services. For example, as we were told during a consultation with the 'Shaping Our Lives' user group:

> *The problem with inspections is that people often don't know the tell-tale signs to look for, and professionals are very good at hiding things. You need to have service users going in and picking things up – they know what to look for.*

3.32   As well as being more attuned to the signs of problems with services because of their own experiences, it is likely that service users are more able to confide in their peers with whom they feel empathy, than with professional inspectors. Box 3.4 gives an example of an innovative approach to engaging service users in this way.

Box 3.4 User involvement in service evaluation and inspection: *the Hampshire Consumer Audit Project*

The Hampshire Consumer Audit Project[*] was established with funding under the Department of Health Community Care Development Programme and run by Southampton Centre for Independent Living. The project recruited and trained 'consumer auditors'. Volunteers needed to be current users of community care services, or carers, and to want to help service users in 'having a say'. The approach was distinguished by an understanding and promotion of the social model of disability, and had the following objectives:

- To develop consumer definitions of outcomes and criteria for their measurement.
- To develop a training and support programme for consumers to undertake independent audits on service outcomes.
- To demonstrate how a focus on the value to consumers can influence commissioning and providing processes.
- To demonstrate a task-focused model of partnership between consumers, health and social services, and the independent sector.

Consumer auditors emphasised a number of strengths of the approach, in particular:

- The independence of the audit, and opportunity for service users to speak to people who understood the issues as 'kindred spirits'.
- Good training and on-going support provided to auditors by the scheme co-ordinators.

*Henwood M. *The Community Care Development Programme: building partnerships for success. An evaluation report to the Department of Health*. London: Department of Health: London, 1998.

3.33 Another example of an innovative approach is that pioneered by The Sainsbury Centre for Mental Health. 'User-focused monitoring' is a model for systematically finding out 'what mental health service users think about living in the community, of their services and of their experiences of being in hospital' (Box 3.5).[25] Significantly, the Sainsbury Centre has successfully developed the model with service users who include people with severe and enduring mental health problems.

Box 3.5 User involvement in service evaluation and inspection: user-focused monitoring *(UFM) of Mental Health Services (Sainsbury Centre for Mental Health)*

- All interviewers were themselves services users. Some of the interviewers were on the top tier of the CPA, 'yet with the right training all completed their interviews and all gained in confidence as a result of doing so'.

- UFM produced 'a different and more open response from their interviewees than professional researchers might have done'.

- All of the evaluations were commissioned by services agencies which were progressive in their approach and committed to user involvement and empowerment.

- Follow-up review indicates that UFM can make a difference, with many changes resulting from the findings.

- Interviewers gain self-esteem from the process; for some, this has led to full-time employment, while others have become more involved in user-focused research.

- UFM is moving into service development by enabling service users to participate in user-led evaluations in their own areas. 'The aim is to concentrate on solutions rather than problems and to ensure that the concerns raised ... are effectively addressed as services evolve'.

Key recommendations arising from UFM include:

- Users should be involved in training all psychiatric and social care professionals.

- Purchasers and providers should facilitate but not control user involvement and empowerment at all levels.

- User involvement in planning and delivering individual care should be for purposes of empowerment not compliance.

- The measurement of the extent of user involvement should be the extent to which users themselves feel involved.

- The complaints of users should be taken seriously. They must not be pathologised or dismissed as symptoms of mental illness.

- There should be systematic user-led evaluations of models of advocacy in mental health.

- Users should be at the centre of the monitoring and evaluation of mental health services.

Source: Rose D. *Users' voices: the perspectives of mental health service users on community and hospital care.* London: The Sainsbury Centre for Mental Health, 2001

The Sainsbury Centre makes, in its own words, 'three large claims' for its approach:

- It empowers service users by giving them real work as interviewers.
- It enables the voices of the most disabled users to be heard and to have an influence on care delivery.
- It provides more accurate and sensitive information about users' experiences of mental health services than do traditional, professional approaches.

3.34   These innovative approaches, and others like them, demonstrate that there is real benefit in promoting active user involvement, and that 'empowerment' can be much more than just a piece of rhetoric. As the Sainsbury Centre initiative points out, such work is in its infancy, and considerable development is needed (including work with other client groups) if UFM is to become more generally accepted. Sainsbury emphasises the importance of the approach as follows:

> *... until recently, mental health service users have not had a voice either in research and evaluation or in influencing care delivery. In an era where we hear much about social exclusion, stigmatisation and empowerment, it is vital to listen to the voices of those who are excluded, stigmatised and disempowered.*[26]

3.35   Expansion of user involvement faces considerable hurdles, not least staff attitudes and perceptions. Those agencies that have become involved with UFM are characterised by a commitment to genuine empowerment, and see themselves at the forefront in such endeavour. Yet even in these positive environments, front-line staff may not share managers' beliefs. Inevitably, it will be harder to promote empowerment in localities that are less than progressive.

Dehumanising treatment and abuse

3.36   Poor quality of service can take many forms, and at the extreme end of the continuum are services in which clients are exploited, neglected, or abused in one way or another. Over the years, there have been many examples of abuse of elderly and other services users. Well-publicised instances have focused largely on cases occurring in residential institutions, and as Biggs *et al.* remark, 'the history of British institutional care is littered with reports prompted by the discovery of mistreatment of elders'.[27] *The Last Refuge*, written by Peter Townsend in 1964, is widely recognised as probably the most influential report on the failings of residential care and the enduring legacy of the workhouse.[28] Further critiques followed from the academic and research community, as well as regular official inquiries into abuse and malpractice in hospitals, care homes, and in the community. These concerned not just elderly people, but also other adult client groups, notably people with learning disabilities, mental health problems, or physical disabilities. The importance of developing an inter-agency response to the abuse of vulnerable adults has been underlined by the Department of Health guidance *No Secrets.*[29]

3.37   The continued existence of poor practices has been highlighted once more in the first report from the Commission for Health Improvement (CHI), and its investigation into the North Lakeland NHS Trust.[30]

3.38   The report identified the development of a culture within the Trust that allowed 'unprofessional, counter-therapeutic and degrading, even cruel, practices to take place'.[31] These included:

- a patient being restrained by being tied to a commode
- patients being denied food
- patients being fed while sitting on commodes
- patients deliberately deprived of clothing and blankets.[32]

3.39   Such practices were unchecked, condoned or even excused when brought to the attention of the trust, and some staff failed to recognise the abuse as unacceptable practice. What is striking about this latest example is the familiarity of the practices identified, and the fact that similar instances have recurred throughout the lifetime of the Welfare State (as indeed they did in the days of its predecessor, the Poor Law regime). The 'whole systems failure' identified by CHI was attributed in large part to the absence of effective management and clinical governance. There is clearly scope for such cultures to emerge within institutional settings. However, there are also opportunities for abuse to take place within the community, particularly where care is provided to people in their own homes, behind closed doors, and in isolation from external gaze. Submissions to the Inquiry echoed such concerns. For example, the Royal College of Physicians remarked:

> *We are certainly concerned about the possibility of abuse of older people. Well documented in hospitals and institutions, it is probably significantly under recognised in care situations at home.*[33]

3.40   Submissions to the Inquiry highlighted relatively little actual abuse of clients, although some examples of assaults under investigation *were* drawn to our attention, as were instances of sexual abuse of service users by care workers. However, the issues on which we sought evidence did not specifically inquire about abuse, and conclusions about the low level of reporting of such cases would be inappropriate. We would also emphasise that there are many different forms of abuse. While physical or sexual assault are the worst examples, there is a range of behaviour that service users experience, and which were frequently identified in submissions to the Inquiry, including:

- patronising staff attitudes and 'talking down' to service users
- controlling behaviour of care staff and removal of decision-making power
- rough handling
- verbal abuse
- racial stereotyping and racist comments
- lack of respect

- financial exploitation and theft.

3.41 We are well aware of the difficulties of identifying abuse, and it is essential that organisational cultures are attuned to recognise instances of abuse, and to have appropriate systems in place for effective response to concerns, allegations and disclosures. New approaches to regulation, enshrined in the Care Standards Act (2000), include measures to improve protection through registration of social care staff, and through the establishment of a list of people considered unsuitable to work with vulnerable adults. Such measures are welcomed, but are not the whole solution. For example, the list can only be effective if it is properly used and providers of care services make appropriate referrals. Moreover, the experience of child protection points to the failures of such systems when there is over-reliance on informal local mechanisms and word of mouth to pass on information or suspicions about individual employees.

3.42 Some evidence of abuse of older clients was provided to the Inquiry by Action on Elder Abuse, based on an analysis of calls made to the Elder Abuse Helpline. The Helpline takes calls from people concerned about others being abused, as well as from people who are themselves victims. Abuse is defined in terms that include not only physical or sexual assault, but also neglect, financial and psychological abuse. We should be cautious of over-extrapolating from the conclusions of this analysis, but some features stand out:

- abuse is *most* likely to take place in a victim's own home
- reports of psychological abuse are nearly twice as common as physical or financial abuse
- physical abuse and neglect are more likely to occur in care settings than in people's own homes
- family members are most likely to be abusers, but *very few of these are direct carers*
- almost 30 per cent of abusers are paid care staff

- although most nurses and care staff are female, two out of five incidents of abuse by staff are perpetrated by males.[34]

3.43 These findings underline the vulnerability of people both in their own homes and in residential/hospital locations. It is essential that adequate safeguards are built into the National Minimum Standards for regulating domiciliary care. The report by Action on Elder Abuse concluded:

> *Callers have given clear indications about the areas of greatest concern to them – for example financial abuse by family members, physical abuse and neglect in care settings, and psychological abuse wherever the older person lives. These concerns now need to be investigated further and research undertaken to identify effective interventions. People who work with this very vulnerable client group need to be trained to ensure that the response from statutory services is one which, while minimising the risk to which they are exposed, respects the adult's right to lead the life they want.[35]*

Driving down costs

3.44 So far, we have highlighted the shortcomings in service quality that have emerged from the analysis. However, there are many ways in which care and support services fail to match up to aspirations of quality. These shortfalls raise questions about the adequacy of resources committed to care and support services in general, and about the impact of commissioning strategies in particular.

3.45 As we outlined in Section 2, the majority of personal support is commissioned, though not provided, by local authorities. A picture emerges from submissions to the Inquiry in which local authority commissioning is increasingly 'bearing down on costs' in the services they pay for, and 'bargaining quality down to a price', leaving very little margin. Taken to the extreme, this is producing a crisis in care provision, with considerable anecdotal evidence to suggest that some providers have been unable to continue supplying a service.[36] It is important to recognise that prior to the introduction of the community care reforms it was understood that this would be a direct consequence of the new role of local authorities. The 1993 inquiry by the House of Commons Health Committee into the funding of community care, for example, observed:

> *In oral evidence, Ministers were keen to persuade us that local authorities will be able to exercise purchasing power as bulk buyers to drive down prices.*[37]

3.46   From early on in the implementation of the community care reforms, the Audit Commission stressed authorities' need to 'strike a balance between commitments and budgeted finance' and to find ways of containing expenditure. In addition to using their purchasing power to control costs, authorities were urged to set needs eligibility criteria 'to allow through just enough people with needs to exactly use up their budget'.[38]

3.47   The power of local authorities to fix prices and negotiate contracts reflects the fact that the social care sector has become in many cases a buyer's market. The social care market has been transformed since the mid-1990s from one in which most services were provided directly by staff employed by the local authority in residential, day care and domiciliary settings, to one in which *most* care workers (more than 60 per cent) are employed in the independent sector.[39] Discussions with the Audit Commission confirmed the trends in the market, which are summarised in Box 3.6.

3.48   A review commissioned from Gowland Taylor Associates by the South and East Economic Development Strategy reinforced such findings with its unequivocal conclusion:

> *The shift from in-house to independent provision has been inextricably linked to reductions in pay and conditions for people delivering care, downward pressure on the price paid for care has been translated into downward pressure on wages.*[40]

We examine issues of employment and remuneration later in this section of the report.

Box 3.6 Cost compression and the social care market

The compression of costs and contract prices in the social care market is reflected by several developments:

- Preoccupation with price not quality.
- Lowered wage levels and conditions of employment to provide price competition.
- Higher eligibility thresholds for service and greater dependency of clients.
- Reduced profit margins leading to:
    - cuts to non-essential front-line services
    - reduced training
    - reduced management support
    - reduced supervision and team meetings.

3.49 How does the picture that emerges from the evidence to the Inquiry compare with other analyses? An important source of information is the programme on the Mixed Economy of Care (MEOC) conducted jointly by the PSSRU and the Nuffield Institute for Health. This ongoing programme has involved mapping the general implementation of the community care legislation, as well as the promotion of a mixed economy of care in a representative sample of 25 English local authority social services departments.[41,42] The MEOC programme has also explored the trade-off between price and quality, and concludes:

> ... *in seeking to drive down costs they might also drive down quality, and our evidence from providers suggests that this has indeed been the result.*[43]

3.50   The MEOC programme has explored the experiences both of providers and of purchasers, and the researchers acknowledge that while some of the concerns expressed by providers are recognised by purchasers as valid, others might be seen as 'exaggerated or are misinterpreting what are, in fact, well-intentioned commissioning strategies'.[44] Nonetheless:

> *Authorities express concerns about quality of care, fearing that the low prices which they themselves are driving down (in pursuit of best value) can only be maintained by independent providers if they employ low-paid, low-skilled staff or cut corners on quality.*[45]

This point was also made in evidence from the Audit Commission to the Royal Commission on Long Term Care, which observed that there was little scope for improving value for money by further cuts to unit costs:

> *... in many areas such cuts may actually reduce quality rather than waste. With the introduction of the minimum wage and with the better targeting of services, unit costs may need to rise if good quality care is to be secured.*[46]

3.51   The consequences of cost control are evident in a number of ways. However, they are reflected particularly in the time pressures faced by care workers in being allocated a fixed amount of time to visit a given number of clients rather than being given autonomy and flexibility in delivering the type of service service users want. The ability to resist demands of service commissioners to undertake short visits (which are disproportionately costly to the provider and are likely to be seen as less satisfying both by care staff and service users) is likely to be greater among larger and more powerful providers.

Submissions to the Inquiry have underlined the practical impact of hurried visits, for example:

> *This results in the relationship between the care worker and the client becoming very task focused – often to the detriment of developing a personal relationship with the client. If a care worker has only one hour in which to perform a number of key tasks, there is little time or scope to talk to the client and develop the human contact side of the relationship.*[47]

The MEOC research has found that providers are less willing to provide short visits (less than 30 minutes). Despite this, almost half of the MEOC sample of providers *are* providing short visits.[48]

3.52   The way in which services are commissioned has a direct bearing, as UKHCA told us:

> *Providers are often not given care plans – even if they exist. This relates to who does the care management on a day to day basis. In home care we don't get a job to do in terms of care – rather we get a time slot and a list of tasks. We are not involved in the actual <u>care</u> of the person – we are just doing things to them. The service commissioners see care as their business. It means that care workers are disenfranchised, and it wastes huge amounts of money because every tiny change has to go back to the commissioner to change the care plan.*[49]

3.53   Again, the extensive evidence of the MEOC research reinforces the findings of the Inquiry. The MEOC 1999 domiciliary care study, for example, indicates providers' concerns 'about not being able to participate in the initial assessments and to utilise their skills and experience'.[50]

3.54   A task-focused approach to the provision of care and support not only undermines the development of supportive, flexible and responsive services, but also makes it virtually impossible to pursue service objectives concerned with maximising independence and preventing physical and psychological decline. This is particularly important because these are precisely the policy objectives being emphasised by Government. It takes longer to provide support to someone in ways that encourage them to exercise independence, than it does to 'do something' to them. A care services that is under pressure to attend to a given number of clients in the shortest possible time will, for example, wash and dress clients rather than help them to manage these things for themselves. This can have deleterious consequences, as this submission to the Inquiry from a person employed as a care assistant observed:

> *Skills are lost where care staff do not have the time or inclination to encourage mobility, hygiene practices, and eating, so clients then need long term care.*[51]

3.55   These pressures add to the stresses on support workers, and can lead them to 'break the rules' in order to deliver the service they believe their clients need. A survey on the management and effectiveness of the home care services carried out by Ian Sinclair and colleagues at the University of York has highlighted such dilemmas:

> *Carers are always moving from one person to another in a time and motion regime, but if you are at all human you realise people are lonely and want to hang on to you. The carers feel responsible, but don't have clout. For example, if there is no food in someone's house and it's not your job to get food, what do you do? If someone has broken their leg, you stay with them. But you won't be paid.*

> *We found that carers were breaking agency rules by taking home users' washing, for example. There is an increasing bureaucratic pressure from the top to tie-down home carers, which impedes their ability to deliver a service with a human face.*[52]

3.56   Commissioning arrangements *can* be structured in ways that give greater autonomy and responsibility to providers to meet users' needs flexibly, and which give scope for negotiating changes to individual care plans. Our analysis, and the views of service users and carers in particular, suggests that this style of commissioning is unusual. Such a style requires a considerable level of trust and maturity in commissioning and provider relationships, and an emphasis not just on cost, and service inputs, but on the outcomes of support for individual service users.

3.57   Evidence from the MEOC programme indicates that, overall, although purchaser/provider relations in social care markets have tended to be adversarial, 'obligational relations built on trust are beginning to develop'.[53] Such relations are characterised by purchasers allowing providers space to get on with the job, and to respond appropriately to changed circumstances 'without the need to get approval for every last detail'. The MEOC team conclude:

> *A task for local authorities is thus to develop strategies which can promote and sustain both competence trust and goodwill trust between trading partners. This might help to contain transaction costs, but has well-known accompanying dangers; trust is a lubricant for transactions, but it must be well-placed and will itself need some monitoring.*[54]

Box 3.7 Towards creative commissioning?

The London Borough of Westminster has developed an approach to commissioning personal care for older people intended to provide greater stability and to necessitate less spot purchasing.

The specification for services required the tendering contractor:

- to ensure the delivery of a reliable, punctual and responsive personal care service to service users
- to enhance the quality of service users' lives
- to ensure that such services are developed in consultation with each service user and their representatives
- to ensure that the provision of the services meets, to a high standard, the needs of service users from different religious, ethnic and cultural backgrounds
- to ensure the service complies with and promotes the fundamental values of privacy, dignity, independence, choice, rights and fulfilment of service users.

Benchmark standards for the quality of service to be delivered were derived from quality standards set out in *Listening to Users of Domiciliary Care Services*.

The reconfiguration of services, focusing on driving up standards, is dependent on developing a solid partnership between the contractors and commissioners. High standards and demanding requirements from contractors are balanced by:

- considerable scope for discretion and flexibility
- guaranteed hours and business, providing stability
- responsibility for *all* care, rather than just for the more difficult or demanding services.

Developing partnership in commissioning

3.58   Since taking office in 1997, the Labour Government has replaced the system of Compulsory Competitive Tendering (CCT) with Best Value. Previously, CCT had applied to a range of services, such as manual services, highway construction, catering and cleaning, and obliged local authorities to undertake competitive tendering. Unlike CCT, which applied only to some services, the duty of Best Value is one that applies to *all* local authority services. Although there is no compulsion to put services out to tender, there is not a presumption that services should be delivered directly by the local authority if other more efficient and effective means are available. The development of Best Value was presented not as an ideological issue, with preconceptions about whether the public, voluntary or private sectors should be preferred providers, but rather that:

> *... these decisions should be based entirely on judgements about best value and optimum outcomes for individual users, and authorities must be able to demonstrate that their arrangements are delivering this.*[55]

3.59   Best Value is intended to ensure that local authorities deliver their services to clear standards of cost *and* quality. However, in practice, there remain concerns over a predominant focus on costs. The Audit Commission's own review of the best value inspection service has made clear that a 'step change in performance' is required to bring in the benefits of the Best Value model, and that few authorities are ambitious enough in what they are seeking to achieve.[56] The 1999 Department of Health report of an inspection of commissioning arrangements for community care services highlighted a 'lack of strategic direction'.[57] A poor approach to commissioning was particularly evident in relation to services for older people, with a lack of services focused on promoting independence or rehabilitation objectives. As the report commented:

It was of concern to find that the traditionally low expectations of older people were matched by those commissioning and providing services to them.[58]

3.60　The lack of strategic planning is associated with shortfalls in the range and type of services available. As already noted, this is shown by the lack of appropriate and relevant services for black and minority ethnic communities, as well as in 'outmoded services which meet neither users' needs nor preferences'.[59] The poor engagement with independent providers in the development of strategic approaches was also underlined by the report:

It was not unusual to find that independent providers were not properly represented in strategic planning arrangements. This was a deficit and at times reflected the adversarial nature of the relationship between some SSDs and the independent sector.[60]

3.61　Even if relationships between commissioners and independent providers are not actively 'adversarial', there is a widespread failure to engage in more productive relationships that allow more autonomy and flexible approaches to meeting needs. There *is* scope for changing this situation (see Box 3.7). The Department of Health inspection reported examples of 'where listening to users and carers and paying attention to their preferences has resulted in dramatically different commissioning practices'.[61] However, the development of responsive and innovative support is far more unusual in services for older people than for those under 65 years. The range of services offered is partly a reflection of what is available locally, but also reflects the general approach to assessment, care planning, monitoring and review. While the Department of Health inspection was critical of social services' failure to engage sufficiently with service users and carers in developing a better understanding of what services are needed, there was less recognition of the implications for commissioning arrangements and market management. We have already highlighted the concordat proposed by the Department of Health as a new approach to managing capacity in the care home sector. This appears to be a recognition of the need to manage capacity and to ensure that services are available when and where required.

3.62 The report commissioned by the South and East Economic Development Strategy has emphasised the need for a shift from competition to partnership in the relations between providers and commissioners, and suggests that 'a core part of partnership building may be the provision of support to the business development of independent providers'.[62] Changing the nature of commissioning is demanding. In addition to improving strategic planning and using a variety of contracts, as the Department of Health recommends,[63] other mechanisms are required if contracts are to be sufficiently flexible, while also ensuring adequate quality assurance and safeguards against unscrupulous providers. For example, submissions to the Inquiry have highlighted the central importance of giving greater care management responsibility to providers if flexibility and responsiveness is genuinely to be encouraged.

Skills and values of care staff

3.63 It is self-evident that the quality of care is fundamentally reliant on the quality of support staff. This has been emphasised by the Chief Inspector's Annual Report, in the observation that 'people's experience of the quality of a service is determined by the quality of the interaction they have with the staff'.[64] Concerns over staff selection, training and management have been major recurrent issues in our Inquiry. There is a spectrum of issues that arises. At one extreme, there are concerns over staff who may pose a direct threat to those they care for, and for whom there are risks of abuse. We will return to this matter when considering regulation issues. More generally, there are issues about staff who may not have the requisite skills and attributes for the work.

3.64 An issue that has arisen repeatedly in the course of the Inquiry is racism expressed between service users and care staff. Service users should have the right to have their race and culture respected and to be provided with appropriate services. Although there may be widespread support for this in principle, *in practice* it may be problematic:

- matching service users with suitable care staff is extremely difficult when there is a shortage of labour

- availability of culturally appropriate services partly depends on recruitment of suitable workers from all cultural and minority ethnic groups, but it depends more fundamentally on the training of *all* care staff to provide appropriate support

- if care work is perceived as low status and even demeaning, some cultural and ethnic groups will not regard it as suitable employment.

3.65   Later in this section, we highlight the over-representation of some black and minority ethnic groups, and the under-representation of some Asian groups and white populations among care staff. It is easy to understand in such situations how the pre-conditions are in place for racist attitudes and prejudices to be expressed. As one of our witnesses remarked:

> *We need to be very careful. There was a home in ... where all the residents were white and the care staff were black, and there were difficulties – older people tend to hold more racist attitudes than younger people. It is tricky; we need to be very sensitive.*[65]

3.66   These *are* difficult issues. If it is poor practice for services to be unable to offer a culturally appropriate service to users, it is surely equally unacceptable to argue for a position of separatism or *de facto* apartheid in services. While some specialised services providing for different black and minority ethnic groups are required, there is a parallel need to ensure that mainstream services are able to offer culturally responsive care. The issue which must be key is that of choice, and ensuring that services are able to meet people's needs and preferences. These preferences are likely to change, and future generations may have quite different attitudes from current ones; they may prefer to use mainstream services rather than ones developed specifically for the black and ethnic minority community.

3.67   Lack of training, or inadequate training, of support staff are major concerns. There are implications not only for client safety, but also for staff welfare. Care and support staff who are inadequately trained will not have the knowledge or skills to undertake safe caring practices. There are questions about the extent to which support workers should have specific skills and knowledge, e.g. in relation to particular conditions and disabilities. However, there is a much bigger question about the absence of generic skills and knowledge, as this submission from the Merseyside Education and Training Consortium to the Inquiry highlights:

> ... *very few organisation offer a comprehensive induction programme for new staff. In effect this means that staff enter the care environment raw, vulnerable and by their ignorance are in themselves at risk, and present a risk to clients.*[66]

Qualifications

3.68   Possession of formal qualifications is in many ways a poor indicator of staff skills. Qualified staff may not necessarily be the most skilled. Conversely, formally unqualified staff may nonetheless have a wealth of skills and knowledge acquired through other experience. Nonetheless, the low level of formal qualification in the care sector is striking, and raises many doubts about the quality of care. A report from the Training Standards Council concludes that the sector struggles to maintain a qualified and experienced workforce. Not only are there long-established 'traditions' of employing untrained staff, particularly in the residential care sector, but crucially, 'there is a correlation between poor workplace practice and poor training'.[67]

3.69   Table 3.1 presents some key data on qualifications, and further information is included in Appendix 1. The fragmented nature of the care sector causes problems in collecting comprehensive data. The Social Services Workforce Survey provides information on those staff directly employed by local authority social services departments. Information on the independent sector is derived from various sample surveys.

Table 3.1 Percentage of social services staff holding qualifications in 1997–9

Qualifications	Area (a)	Area (b)	Home care	Day care	Resid- ential care	Special needs	Total
Professional social work	37.3	95	0.3	7.1	6.2	24.0	22.9
Management (including NVQ assessor)	2.9	14.7	1.7	5.1	4.7	6.2	5.7
Nursing	0.9	0.0	0.9	2.0	2.2	3.2	1.2
S/NVQ	6.7	0.0	3.2	10.1	6.6	4.4	4.6
Other	13.6	0.0	1.7	13.5	12.4	19.0	6.5
Total qualified	56.5	95.0	6.5	42.5	26.4	47.2	36.4
Total not qualified	43.5	5.0	93.5	57.5	73.6	52.8	63.6
Numbers in the sample	6,120	45,217	78,571	31,676	63,967	1,502	222,053

Source: Social Services Workforce Survey, 1999

Area (a): covers occupational therapists (OT), OT assistants and community workers. Area (b): senior directing staff, assistant directors, team leaders, assistant team leaders, and field social workers and care managers.

3.70   As Table 3.1 shows, just over one in three social services staff are qualified, and two-thirds of qualified staff hold a professional social work qualification. Home care staff are notable for their low level of qualification, which at more than 90 per cent is far greater than for any other area of social services support work. Moreover, it is apparent that changing this situation will be demanding: in the same period, only 6.4 per cent of social services home care staff were studying for qualifications. This was the lowest proportion of all social services staff, and runs against the trend evident for other staff where a low level of qualification was associated with a *greater likelihood* of being in current training (Figure 3.1).

Figure 3.1 Proportion of social services staff unqualified, and proportion currently studying for qualification 1997–9

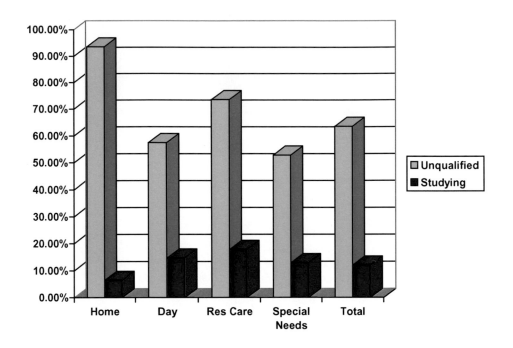

Source: Social Services Workforce Survey, 1999

3.71   Higher proportions of home care staff appear to be qualified in the independent sector than in local authority home care services. However, these findings must be interpreted cautiously since information on the independent sector relies heavily on self-selecting survey responses, and respondents may not be representative of all employees. Thus, for example, UKHCA carried out a national survey of home care staff in 2000 to try and fill the gap in the data and understanding of the independent sector. The survey found nearly one-third (31 per cent) of home care respondents held and/or were studying for a qualification. However, these figures are considerably higher than other estimates suggest, and may overstate the level of qualification across the sector overall.

3.72   Nonetheless, the UKHCA findings are of interest, not least because they contribute knowledge about a sector where relatively little is known. Even if the figures on training and qualification levels in the independent sector *are* robust, there remain questions about whether the level of qualification is rising, and how long it will be before most employees are qualified. The UKHCA survey also found younger staff more likely to hold qualifications than staff aged over 30 (see Appendix 1). Whether this will have a significant effect in raising qualification levels over time depends to a large extent on maintaining a supply of younger staff, and ensuring that they remain in the sector. We return to questions of recruitment and retention at a later stage.

What skills are needed?

3.73   The training needs of both health and social care staff have shifted in recent times, reflecting changes that have taken place in the respective roles and responsibilities of these workers. Social care staff are increasingly undertaking personal care tasks that until recently would have been viewed as the responsibility of the district or community nurse. Since 1993 and the advent of the community care reforms, there has been an accelerated shift away from the traditional model of the 'home help' service, and towards the model of home care that is focused less on domestic support than on personal care and assistance. Indeed, much of the controversy surrounding paying for long-term care has highlighted the distinction between nursing care and personal care. This is often more apparent than real, and much of what is classified as 'personal care', and therefore the responsibility of social services, is indistinguishable in common sense terms from 'nursing care', which is considered to be an NHS responsibility.[68]

3.74   The changing nature of home care is at the heart of many of the issues around quality of care and support. It is precisely *because* there has been a shift towards more personal care that different concerns over quality have come to the fore. The quality of support is of less significance, and potential risk, when it is concerned primarily with housework, than when it is about support with personal, and often highly intimate, quasi-nursing tasks. In such circumstances, the quality of the relationship with the support worker, and the level of skill and knowledge which that person has, become extremely significant.

3.75   The emphasis on training the social care workforce and on the expansion of qualifications is not only about the development of technical competence. The UKHCA survey of home care staff asked about experiences of training undertaken in the preceding 12 months. The most frequently identified categories of training were:

- moving and handling (39 per cent)
- first aid (13 per cent)
- food and hygiene (6 per cent)
- health and safety (5 per cent).[69]

A wide range of other categories of training were also identified, but these were mentioned by very small proportions of staff. For example:

- awareness of dementia or Alzheimer's disease (3 per cent)
- awareness of other special needs groups, such as learning disabilities, physical disabilities, mental health needs, sensory impairment, HIV (3 per cent)
- awareness of particular conditions and illness, such as diabetes, epilepsy, stroke, cancer, etc. (2 per cent).

3.76   The very characteristics of staff that service users value highly, such as understanding, compassion, awareness of needs and requirements, etc., are the areas that are apparently least likely to be the focus of training. The concentration is overwhelmingly on the statutory aspects of training that must be undertaken as a bare minimum for induction purposes. However, some submissions to the Inquiry demonstrated that it is possible to address wider issues in training. The Mental Health Foundation, for example, has developed a certificate in community mental health care to do just this (Box 3.8).

Box 3.8 Developing new qualifications in care: *The Certificate in Community Mental Health Care*

The certificate was developed to tackle the 'piecemeal approach' to training and to ensure that a single course could provide comprehensive coverage of the core knowledge, skills and attitudes needed by practitioners to deliver effective and safe client-centred services.

The qualification is aimed at staff, volunteers, service users and carers without a professional qualification in mental health, but who are involved in the delivery of mental health services. The Certificate covers 11 units:

- mental health problems and their impact
- management of treatment approaches
- working with people with mental health problems
- legislation, policies and mental health services
- care planning
- communication and relationships with service users
- promoting independence
- supporting individuals with relationships
- enabling people to manage change
- team and joint working
- working with carers and support groups.

Further information: www.mentalhealth.org.UK/certificate

Similarly, the Joseph Rowntree Foundation has established a Certificate in Care aimed at bridging the gap between health and social care training (Box 3.9).

Box 3.9 Developing new qualifications in care: *The Joseph Rowntree Foundation (JRF) Certificate in Care*

The JRF Certificate in Care was launched at the end of 1998. With its focus on bridging health and social care training, it is intended to equip care staff with the skills and knowledge base necessary to enable the people in their care to fulfil their potential for an independent and dignified quality of life.

The JRF Certificate has been developed by the Joseph Rowntree Foundation and the University of Lincolnshire and Humberside, and promotes itself as *the* professional qualification for care staff. The Certificate can be converted to an NVQ Level 4 in Care, and it addresses:

- physical sciences
- social behavioural sciences
- problem solving
- study skills
- teamworking skills
- activities related to specific care interventions.

Further information: www.jrf.org.UK/housingtrust/certificateincare

---

3.77   The lack of training in the principles and values of personal care was identified repeatedly in submissions to the Inquiry. For example, the Royal National Institute for the Deaf (RNID) told us how deaf people frequently identify 'poor attitudes' on the part of support workers:

> *... they indicate that service providers are impatient and inconsiderate and that they lack confidence in communicating with deaf and hard of hearing people. This is caused by insufficient training and reflects*

society's attitudes. It is well appreciated in the field of residential care that service providers sometimes assume that older people who do not respond appropriately or quickly are confused or suffering from dementia. However, their lack of response may simply be caused by their communication difficulties, especially if service providers are unaware of this possibility.[70]

3.78   Many other comments reflect similar concerns. The Stroke Association for example remarked to us that:

... there are many workers visiting people with stroke who have no insight into the problems associated with the disability and this is likely to be the case for other disabilities.[71]

The Alcohol Problems Advisory Service also remarked:

Care workers seem unsure about how to recognise problematic alcohol use and are ignorant of issues relating to the client's safety.[72]

3.79   The skills and knowledge that care and support workers may lack in these examples are concerned with the understanding of particular conditions and circumstances. Such issues can be particularly problematic in respect of conditions that are relatively unusual (such as Parkinson's disease, or Progressive Supranuclear Palsy). However, as pointed out in Section 2 of our report, demographic pressures and an emphasis on supporting people in the community, wherever possible, are contributing to an increasing complexity of needs, which care staff must understand. There are also wider concerns about the lack of understanding or awareness of principles of independent living. These issues have also been amplified in submissions to the Inquiry, for example:

Vulnerable adults are often not given the freedom to use physical space, express emotional feelings, make social relationships or participate in cultural and/or spiritual activities that might enhance their lives or strengthen their sense of identity.[73]

3.80   The denial of opportunities to exercise independence and choice, to be afforded privacy, or to be supported in taking appropriate risks, typically arises when care and support workers are concerned with 'looking after' clients rather than with acting in an enabling role. Qualitative research with service users has identified similar concerns, emphasising, for example, workers who are over-authoritarian and controlling in their interaction. As this mental health service user told the 'Shaping Our Lives' group:

> *They think that they are the professionals and you are not even a normal person. They believe that they have the authority to tell you how to run your life. That type of professional doesn't help you, they make you worse.*[74]

3.81   It is often said that good carers are 'born not made'. Up to a point, this may be so, but there is much that training *can* (and must) do to impart the skills that high-quality staff need, and to inculcate the values which should inform care and support. Staff need to appreciate the importance to service users of retaining independence and autonomy, and of having control and choice, but there are also more fundamental and basic issues about respect and courtesy. The qualitative literature on the views of service users consistently emphasises dissatisfaction with 'patronising' attitudes, and with lack of respect for privacy and confidentiality. In the consultation undertaken by 'Shaping Our Lives', a service user with learning difficulties made the following comment:

> *Two care workers used to come to look after me sometimes. They just talked to each other all the time. Sometimes I talked to them and they didn't even look at me.*[75]

3.82   Similar issues were identified in submissions to the Inquiry, and in our wider consultation processes (see Appendices 2 and 3). It is important to note that many service users have nothing but praise for their support workers. However, there remain concerns about the poor skills and attitudes of a minority. For example, in the course of the Inquiry's consultation with service users, the following comments were made:

>   *They need to treat us as human beings, not as lumps of meat.*

>   *I don't understand why these people go into this work, because they don't care.*

>   *I've been psychologically abused and bullied with the threat that if I don't toe the line I will lose service support.*

>   *People go into these professions to come and 'look after' you. It isn't about empowerment and enabling people to live independent lives – there are major training issues there. And you have to fight for your rights all the time and struggle against that culture.*

3.83   In some situations the problem is not one of a lack of training, but of inappropriate or irrelevant training. The independent living movement, for example, which has pushed for Direct Payments and for the use of personal assistants who can work to the user's specification, has emphasised that service users are the best people to train support staff.

3.84   As noted previously, staff can be skilled in many ways, and this can also be true in the absence of formal qualifications. As TOPSS (the National Training Organisation for social care) points out in its national training strategy:

>   *The existence of people with qualifications is not necessarily the same as the availability of skills in the workplace. We have treated unqualified staff as a key indicator of skill gaps for the purpose of this*

analysis as there is no other obvious measure. Substantial resources go on 'in house' training of short duration and with no linkage to career pathways or qualifications. TOPSS England recognises and values the benefits of unaccredited 'in house' training and the skills and experiences contributed by many unqualified staff to the delivery of quality services.[76]

3.85 Nonetheless, the way forward will be conditional on the adoption of National Occupational Standards, with all new entrants to the workforce receiving structured induction. TOPSS is clear that the training and development needs, both of existing staff and of new entrants to the workforce, 'will place substantial demands on management, practice and support staff'. We agree that this will certainly be the case, but our evidence overwhelmingly underlines the importance of pursuing such a strategy if the workforce *is* to be able to meet the modernisation agenda in care. We return to these issues when considering regulation.

Employment

3.86 At the heart of many of the problems with care and support are major challenges in the recruitment and retention of staff. It is becoming increasingly difficult to recruit staff, and in some areas this has reached a crisis point with home care agencies, for example, unable to continue providing a service. Difficulties in recruitment and retention of workers have direct consequences for the quality of services, particularly when shortages of staff force an unplanned reliance on agency staff. The causes of this situation are complex and multifactorial. Submissions to the Inquiry have identified:

- overall shortages in the labour market reflecting a strong and growing economy
- multiple competitors for a limited pool of workers
- shortage of people with the right skills and/or qualities
- apparent low status of care work, reflected in poor pay and conditions
- no career pathways or security.

3.87   The difficulties produced by these circumstances were emphasised repeatedly in submissions to the Inquiry. For example, as the Association for Residential Care observed:

> *With extended periods of staff shortages it is difficult to maintain the quality of support; hard to offer much one to one quality time with individuals and hard to maintain staff morale. With some supermarkets offering £8 per hour to stack shelves overnight it is hard to attract staff to a complex and often stressful job for much less money. In some parts of the country providers say that the only people applying for vacancies are those that McDonalds and Tesco have already rejected, and if employed they come with high numeracy and literacy training needs, quite apart from any induction training and values based training needs.*[77]

3.88   Evidence from the MEOC research programme has similarly documented the problems of providers in recruiting suitable staff. Not only do three-quarters of respondents report problems with recruitment, but *nearly one-third rejected at least half of their applicants as unsuitable.*[78]

3.89   The report of the Joint Reviews of human resource performance by the Audit Commission and Social Services Inspectorate (SSI), pointed out that the projected workforce in social care requires continued and faster recruitment growth in a static employment market in order to offset turnover and retirement.[79] Moreover, the difficulties are made worse by a very similar recruitment problem in teaching, nursing and related professions, which are all competing for the same potential recruits. In such an environment, recruitment is very likely to become more difficult. We have referred previously to the changing nature of care and support work that reflects the downward substitution of professional tasks. Thus, a proportion of the work previously undertaken by doctors is now undertaken by nurses; while traditional nursing work is typically being undertaken by health care assistants and personal care staff. This has been one approach to dealing with particular skills shortages.

However, in this shifting hierarchy of the professions, the only group below care and support staff to whom further delegation and substitution can take place is that of volunteers.

3.90 The Joint Review confirmed other evidence in finding staff recruitment to be a problem in most councils. Planning to attract the right people requires a more strategic approach to workforce planning. The review highlighted the importance of councils addressing the workforce requirements for social care *in the voluntary and private sectors*, as well as in the local authority arena. Strategic planning, it is argued:

> *... must be related to longer term community needs, service objectives and local economic development strategies.*[80]

The report to the South and East Economic Development Agency has similarly emphasised the need to support and develop a learning culture, by valuing training and linking successes to both practical and financial benefits.[81]

3.91 A high staff turnover can be extremely problematic, not only in necessitating constant re-training of the workforce, but in undermining any attempt to ensure continuity of care and support to service users. The Recruitment and Retention Survey in social services and in independent sector residential and nursing homes estimated the turnover of local authority home care staff at 16 per cent, and at almost 22 per cent in independent sector care homes (see Appendix 1). Some turnover reflects staff moving on to other types of care work, but there is also a turnover of staff moving completely out of the care sector. The UKHCA survey found that 37 per cent of respondents had been care workers for less than two years. However, alongside this picture of high turnover, there is also paradoxically a large proportion of staff who remain for a long period; the UKHCA survey found 30 per cent of staff had been in the care sector for at least five years.

3.92   There are significant differences between the public and independent care sectors, and in-house providers have a lower staff turnover than the independent sector. In London, there is evidence of considerable 'churning' in the home care market (i.e. a high level of staff movement between various providers in response to marginal changes in pay and conditions of employment, or in the availability of employment because of changing contracts).[82] In a competitive market and a thriving economy, unattractive employment is less acceptable than in conditions of high unemployment. Not surprisingly, care providers facing the greatest recruitment problems are those in areas of economic growth.

The care occupations labour force

3.93   An understanding of the current labour force is important in considering likely developments. The analysis commissioned by the Inquiry from the PSSRU (see Appendix 1) identified the 'care occupations sub-sample' from the Labour Force Survey (incorporating care assistants, social workers, nurses, occupational therapists, nursing assistants and auxiliaries, and cleaners and domestics). Table 3.2 summarises the age breakdown of this sub-sample, alongside data on home care staff derived from the UKHCA survey.

Table 3.2 The care labour force by age

Age group (years)	Labour force survey sub-sample	UKHCA home care staff
Under 30	19%	19%
30–39	24%	24%
40–49	26%	25%
50+	31%	32%

3.94   The findings from the two surveys are virtually identical, and indicate that the workforce is a relatively mature one. The workforce is also predominantly female (around 90 per cent), and employed on a part-time basis. Information on the ethnic composition of the workforce comes from the social services workforce surveys. A comparison between these findings and information for the working population covered by the Labour Force Survey indicates that:

- black Africans, black Caribbeans, and other groups of black staff are *over-represented* in social services employment compared with their representation in the working population overall (5.6 per cent compared with 2.3 per cent), while Bangladeshi, Indian and Pakistani people are *under-represented* (2.6 per cent compared with 5.7 per cent).

- white people in social services employment are also *under-represented* compared to the working age population overall (89 per cent compared with 93 per cent).

3.95   The UKHCA survey found the proportion of domiciliary care workers from ethnic minority backgrounds was closer to the proportions for the working age population overall. However, these figures are likely to be an underestimate, given low response rates to the UKHCA survey from London and other metropolitan areas in which the proportion of home care workers from ethnic minority backgrounds is know to be higher (see Appendix 1).

3.96   As the UKHCA survey makes clear, the social care market is highly fragmented and localised. Difficulties in recruitment and retention vary geographically, and problems are particularly acute in the South East, where unemployment is low and there is plenty of choice for employees seeking part-time flexible employment.

3.97   Wage levels for care and support work are generally low, though there are significant variations between areas, and between different types of care work.

- The Labour Force Survey indicates that the mean gross hourly pay for care assistants and attendants in 1998 was £4.57.

- Private nursing and residential homes generally pay lower wage rates than local authority homes (the majority of private care homes were paying *less than £4.00 per hour*).

- A survey conducted for UNISON in December 2000, found average pay of in-house home care staff to be £5.24 per hour.[83]

3.98   We have referred previously to some of the consequences that the privatisation of care services has had in driving down service costs and suppressing wage levels. Although staff who transfer from the public to the private sector initially have their pay and conditions protected, there is evidence that this erodes over time. In particular, new staff do *not* enter employment with this protection, and a two-tier workforce emerges between transferred staff and new employees.[84]

3.99   There are major questions about raising levels of pay and improving terms and conditions of employment. This is likely to be necessary to increase the competitiveness of the sector in the labour market, *and* to raise the status of the work. It is clear that low pay continues to characterise the sector, and exploits the loyalty and commitment of many staff. The driving down of costs contributes to low wages, and without realistic pricing of contracts, rises in National Minimum Wages will continue to squeeze some independent providers out of the market. As we have indicated, the care workforce is an ageing one, and without appealing to new and younger employees, more acute problems in recruitment and retention can be predicted, as the public sector union UNISON remarked in a submission to the Inquiry:

> *It is already widely acknowledged that we are facing a growing recruitment crisis amongst care and support workers. People do earn more on a supermarket check-out than as a care worker ... As we approach full employment, unless we can rebuild the sense of pride in public services* <u>*and*</u> *offer better wages and improved training opportunities, then there is no serious prospect of raising the standards of the services we deliver.*[85]

3.100   The UKHCA survey has also emphasised the problems. It is expected that the growth in the social care workforce overall will continue at 2.5 to 3 per cent a year, and home care at an even faster rate, but this has to take place in the context of an overall labour force expected to grow by less than 0.5 per cent a year. In such circumstances, competition for a limited pool of labour can only intensify. It is expected that there will be particular difficulties in recruiting women in the 35 to 44-year-old age group in light of other demographic and socio-economic trends. As the TOPSS National Training Strategy has remarked, the sector will need to consider 'whether to recruit from a significantly younger age group and men of all ages to fill jobs, bearing in mind that both these groups will continue to fall in the overall workforce pool'.[86]

Improving recruitment and retention?

3.101 The impending sense of crisis in the situation of the social care workforce is unavoidable. The Chief Inspector of Social Services has observed that:

> *The entire modernisation of the social services is in jeopardy without a fully staffed, well trained workforce to take forward the improvements that we are making.*[87]

However, this objective of achieving 'a fully staffed, well trained workforce' is incompatible with the realities of the labour market in general, and of the social care market in particular, *unless there is major change.*

3.102 The Audit Commission's analysis has underlined the importance of councils improving their 'people management' skills as the key to high-quality services. It is undoubtedly true that social services departments *do* need to have effective human resource policies to recruit and retain high-quality staff. However, it is equally clear that these issues need to be addressed throughout the independent sector, as the major provider of support services.

3.103 Poor pay is clearly a major factor in recruitment and retention difficulties. Indeed, poor conditions may be responsible for deterring entrants of a higher calibre, and for encouraging a culture in which poor standards of conduct and service are tolerated or condoned. In situations of poor supply, employers may be less rigorous in their recruitment practices than would otherwise be the case; personnel who have been sacked or who have been suspected of poor practice may be able to continue to work in the care sector.

3.104 The image of care and support is one of low-status manual work. It does not reflect the realities of the highly skilled support that is often required. As Lesley Bell has commented:

> *Domiciliary care is still seen as just a matter of cleaning and shopping, but the work is very demanding, both physically and emotionally. Domiciliary workers are dealing with very vulnerable people in their own homes and they have to cope with considerable needs and dependencies with very little support. Why would you want to do all this if you can go and work at Tescos?*[88]

3.105 The motivation of providers, and of individual care workers, are complex. Clearly, factors other than financial reward must be significant. The MEOC research has explored providers' backgrounds and expressed motivations. It identified the three most important motives identified by independent sector providers as:

- meeting the needs of older people
- professional accomplishment
- developing or using skills and expertise.[89]

Maximising income and profit was *least* frequently identified as a motivation. Interviews with care staff indicated a similar pattern of motivation.

3.106 Increasing the attractions of home care employment, and related fields of support work, will require moves to raise the status of the work and to address training and staff development. This may help recruit people who wish to enter the care field because they have a genuine interest in caring work, and see it as a vocation. However, it may be unrealistic to imagine it will address the interests of a wider group of employees for whom it is 'just a job' from which they will move on sooner or later. This may be the nettle that has to be grasped: the challenge in recruitment and retention must be to appeal to more of the former group and fewer of the latter.

3.107 There is a vicious circle operating. Care and support is seen as low-status work and is typically characterised by poor pay and prospects. Because of this, recruits to the work are usually people with few labour market choices, which in turn reinforces and perpetuates the low status. As a care assistant writing in the journal *Community Care* observed:

> *Whether you work for a social services department or in the private sector it appears that care assistants do not seem to be held in very high regard – by the public in general and by some senior management in social care ... Is it because we do the job that seems to fill so many with disgust?*[90]

3.108 The fact that there *are* pockets of practice in which recruitment and retention are more successful may point to possible ways forward. Boxes 3.10 and 3.11 explore some of the experiences of greater success that were drawn to the attention of the Inquiry.

3.109 Other experiences indicate some of the features that may contribute to easier recruitment and retention. In giving oral evidence to the Inquiry, Julia Twigg highlighted the following:

- innovative schemes can recruit higher quality workers
- care work has a different status for workers in transition
- the majority of care workers have limited employment choices
- there is considerable autonomy for individual care workers
- the work is stressful, but does contain intrinsic rewards.[91]

Box 3.10 Raising the status of home care in Bradford

In Bradford, a request for 'corporate workwear' came directly from home care assistants themselves. The workwear is seen to present a professional image of the home care service. It raised the status of both the service, and of the social services department more broadly, to something similar to that of health care colleagues. Home care staff reported that being seen as 'professional' was important to them. For Bradford social services, the introduction of corporate workwear was an opportunity to improve service consistency – staff would look the same, and services users and their carers should be able to expect similar standards of service. Staff from minority ethnic communities were consulted about the garments, and the range reflects the cultural diversity of staff members.

Following the introduction of the workwear, home care workers have made positive comments such as:

'I get more respect from people', and *'I felt professional wearing the garments'*, and *'people in the chemist, and GP receptionists seemed to react differently to me'*.

Twigg's research on home care in the London labour market found that the independent sector was drawing on the same limited pool of workers as the local authority, but in addition:

> *... they recruited strongly among transient workers: young, mostly white, women from countries like New Zealand, Zimbabwe, Australia, funding their travel in Europe by doing care work. In the racialised workforce of care, these young women are able to capitalise on their cultural capital as white and middle class.*[92]

3.110 Other groups of 'transitional workers' attracted to care work were also identified:

> *The voluntary sector bathing service ... had a mixed group of staff that reflected the capacity of innovative schemes to recruit higher quality staff. A number of their care workers ... had degrees and many were transitional workers, doing bathing work on their way to something else, sometimes in the care sector, for example, graduate nursing or social work. They also recruited people working in the arts who were putting together work but the real focus of whose lives was elsewhere.*[93]

As we have noted above, geographical variations in the labour market are significant, and the innovative approaches described here were a reflection of the particular circumstances in London, which may not be easily replicated elsewhere.

Box 3.11 Easier recruitment and retention?

In the course of the Inquiry, certain areas of support were identified as ones in which it is relatively easier to attract and retain care and support staff. These include:

- housing support
- mental health support
- AIDS and HIV support.

It is possible that there are greater intrinsic satisfactions in working with these client groups, and opportunities for more fulfilling work. In housing and mental health support, for example the role is likely to differ from that of someone primarily supporting an older person. There will be less emphasis on personal *care* than on enabling independence and personal achievement.

However, there is anecdotal evidence that the challenges of recruitment and retention in these areas may have been delayed rather than avoided altogether.

The field of AIDS and HIV provides a further example. Success in recruiting and retaining high-quality and committed support workers has been a distinctive feature of such services. Unlike many other areas of support, this may reflect a tendency for the homosexual community to care for its own. Services for AIDS/HIV were originally set up by homosexual men because of the absence of any appropriate support. Changes in AIDS/HIV are having consequences for services and volunteer recruitment; the lower profile given to the issue than in the past is believed to contribute to a lower public awareness of needs, and a lack of understanding that it is not exclusively a male homosexual issue. With new medication regimes, people are surviving much longer with AIDS/HIV, and have lesser needs for personal *care*, than for support in dealing with associated problems (e.g. mental health needs and depression, and dealing with personal debt).

Violence against social care staff

3.111   In addition to the problems of low pay and poor conditions of employment previously identified, there is the additional problem of violence. A National Task Force on Violence Against Social Care Staff was established by the Secretary of State for Health, Frank Dobson MP, in September 1999. The Task Force reported in January 2001.[94] Research conducted to explore the impact of violence in the social care workforce found:

> *... a widespread feeling of both lack of recognition and lack of appreciation for the people and the work involved in social care.*[95]

Staff believed the lack of recognition and appreciation to be reflected in the attitudes of the general public, of the media, and of other professionals. They reported feeling undervalued and underpaid, and saw the two as intrinsically linked:

> *For me it is an issue that comes of finance because they can't afford to give the staff the appropriate training, they can't afford to fully staff us all the time, staff aren't getting paid enough for the environment they are in ... so you are not getting the quality of staff, and staff that are any good move on and out.*[96]

3.112   The Task Force emphasised three reasons why a reduction of risk and incidence of violence and abuse must be pursued:

- responsibility for the health, safety and welfare of staff
- improved outcomes for service users
- improved efficiency of each employer's business.[97]

The National Task Force defined violence against workers as:

... incidents where persons are abused, threatened or assaulted in circumstances relating to their work, involving an explicit or implicit challenge to their safety, well being or health. This definition is taken to include verbal abuse or threat, threatening behaviour, any assault (and any apprehension of unlawful violence) and serious or persistent harassment, and extends from what may seem to be minor incidents to serious assault and murder, and threats against the worker's family.[98]

3.113   In aiming to reduce violence and the threat of violence, the Task Force recognised that there are no simple answers, and that a combination of factors must be addressed including:

- the working environment
- the way work is organised
- working practices
- service user expectations
- public perceptions of social care workers and the job they do.

On the matter of public perceptions, the Task Force comments:

Frontline workers are quite sure that the low public esteem in which they are held encourages or at least disinhibits violent behaviour. There is good evidence that the media creates a perception of social care workers which is much more negative than is the actual perception of those who use their services. We know that those involved with the establishment of the General Social Care Council are committed to improving public esteem for the workforce and we see that as an important responsibility of the new body.[99]

The Task Force also laid responsibility with Ministers for ensuring they should use their public influence 'to encourage a proper valuing of social work and social care work'.

3.114 One of the key principles established by the Task Force is that service users have responsibilities as well as rights, and one such responsibility is not to abuse care staff. This is an important principle that others have also endorsed.[100] UNISON has developed guidelines on handling racial harassment, and these also emphasise the vital role of management in demonstrating a commitment through a clear policy statement and established procedures for responding to incidents and allegations.[101] Work by the Continuing Care Conference on developing a framework contract between home care providers and service users has similarly argued the rights and responsibilities equilibrium (Box 3.12).

Box 3.12 Rights and responsibilities in care

As a service user you have a right to:

- courtesy from your carers
- confidentiality about your personal circumstances
- privacy
- be treated equally and to have your religion, culture, etc., respected
- have your wishes respected
- know how to complain, and to whom if you are not satisfied.

You have a responsibility to:

- let them know if you do not need the service at any time
- pay the charges for the services promptly
- respect the cultural differences of others, including those caring for you by not discriminating on the grounds of race or gender or religion
- ensure that any suitable equipment and/or materials are available for the home care worker if that forms part of your agreed service
- ensure that you and your suppliers are adequately covered by public liability insurance
- provide a reasonably safe working environment for the providers.

Source: Continuing Care Conference. *Framework contract between domiciliary care provider and service user.* London: The Continuing Care Conference, 1998

3.115 Care workers involved in the research undertaken by the Task Force on violence in social care also believed that displaying notices in the workplace about intolerance of violence was an important step, not least for the symbolic messages that it conveyed. There was low awareness among these staff that the Department of Health had established a Task Force, and a degree of cynicism about anything that might be achieved as a result.[102] The Task Force has posted many resource materials on its web site, including a model statement aimed at achieving mutual respect between those using services and those working in them, which could be adapted for use in areas where there is a potential risk (Box 3.13).

Box 3.13 Code of conduct

The Task Force suggests that a card or notice, with an audio version for non-readers and visually impaired people, could be given to everyone. Each workplace might adapt it a little, but should not make it long or difficult to read. The following Code of Conduct could be considered for service users and staff.

Welcome to ...

To ensure safety and respect for everyone who uses or works in this service:

- no physical violence
- no verbal abuse or threats
- no racial or sexual harassment
- no sexual relationships between workers and service users
- no alcohol misuse
- no street drugs

are tolerated.

http://www.doh.gov.UK/violencetaskforce/environment.htm

Regulation and training

3.116   As we outlincd in Section 2, regulation is the linchpin of the Government's policy for securing wholesale improvements in care and support. The 1998 White Paper, *Modernising Social Services*, acknowledged the widespread criticisms that 'the present regulatory arrangements are incomplete and patchy'. It also signalled the intention to 'replace them with a system that is modern, independent and dependable', and specifically to:

- put in place new systems for ensuring that when people receive care, 'it is safe and of high quality, that they have adequate living standards if they are in care homes, and that the staff on whom they rely have the training, skills and standards that are necessary for the work that they do'

- create a new General Social Care Council (GSSC) to be responsible for regulating the training of social workers; set conduct and practice standards for all social services staff; and 'register those in the most sensitive areas'

- develop a new training strategy centred around a new National Training Organisation for social care staff.[103]

3.117   The establishment of the GSSC, which would *for the first time regulate social care personnel,* was argued to be necessary in order to:

- improve public protection

- raise the quality of services and improve performance

- give proper recognition to the vocational commitment of the workforce.[104]

3.118   The Care Standards Act (2000) subsequently introduced the primary legislation required to implement these changes. The Act is potentially one of the most significant pieces of legislation ever produced in the arena of social care. The main purpose of the Act is to reform and bring into regulation care services in England and Wales, ranging from residential and nursing homes, domiciliary care agencies and independent health care services, to children's services. For the first time, local authorities will be required to meet the same standards as independent sector providers. The Act is a critical part of what the Government describes as 'the modernisation imperative' in social services, and is a key component of a wider quality strategy. The central concern is to 'set in place a national framework to promote excellence'. The Act is intended to ensure that health and social services will be safe; meet proper quality standards, and will be delivered by skilled and competent staff wherever they are provided, and *whether by staff in the public or independent sectors*. The Act also established the National Care Standards Commission (which was also one of the core recommendations made by the Royal Commission on Long Term Care). The Commission is to have a broad remit, and will be responsible for regulating and inspecting the full range of care services. The Commission must also keep the Secretary of State generally informed on the provision, availability and quality of services, and may make recommendations about changes to National Minimum Standards with a view to seeking improvement in the quality of services.

3.119 The Care Standards Act puts quality on the agenda of social care as never before. Much is promised. The machinery is being put in place to address regulation, safety, and raise standards. The key question that has to be asked is whether the new modernisation agenda and the strategy for quality in social care *will* deliver what it promises. Some commentators may argue that it is too soon to begin to make such judgements, and undoubtedly the changes will take time to deliver their objectives. The Act provides a framework for radical change and, if carried forward, is capable of addressing many of the quality concerns raised in this report. However, the more fundamental question is whether the policy framework that is being put in place *will* produce the desired results, or whether additional strategies are required in order to tackle a wider range of issues.

Regulation and registration

3.120   The Care Standards Act provides for the GSSC in England (and for comparable bodies in Scotland, Wales and Northern Ireland) to regulate the conduct and practice of social care workers. Each of the four councils will be independent, but a high level of co-operation is expected in order to avoid problems with differential levels of protection for service users in different parts of the UK.[105] The new councils will be responsible for:

- registering social care workers
- setting standards in social care work
- regulating the education and training of social workers.

Registration of social care workers will not take place immediately, but rather will occur incrementally, by occupational group. Registration will start with those groups among whom qualification levels are highest, i.e. social workers. Registration of social care workers will not take place until an (as yet, unspecified) critical mass of qualification level is reached. In England, the next target group for early registration is that of residential child care workers, for whom training to NVQ level 3 is a priority to ensure they are among the early registrants with the GSCC.[106]

3.121   Submissions to the Inquiry have identified concerns over this incremental approach. UNISON has observed that while the Government has made the drive to raise standards the central feature of its modernisation programme, 'the tools to bring about this desirable end result are not available to the Government'.[107] The delay in extending registration requirements will hold back the process, and UNISON argues that 'a massive investment in training opportunities is a pre-requisite for raising standards'.

3.122   Alternative approaches have been proposed. In 1992, the National Institute for Social Work (NISW) argued the case to the Conservative Secretary of State for Health for the establishment of a General Social Services Council, and addressed the question of registration. A register of people working in social care would essentially establish and maintain public confidence, moreover:

> *The major concern of the Action Group is that registration must quickly and effectively assist in the protection of the most vulnerable members of the public through the registration of those who are in a position of immediate and considerable power over such individuals.*[108]

3.123   As NISW went on to argue, entry to professional registers is based upon the acquisition of a relevant qualification. As we have seen, the majority of the social care workforce does not hold such a qualification, and:

> *... in order to achieve the aim of protecting the public, it would be impossible to exclude this majority, which would be the consequence of a register based upon qualification alone.*[109]

3.124   Access to, and resources to support, training will not allow the emergence of a qualified workforce to occur in the near future. The NISW Action Group proposed an alternative strategy that would establish a limited register of those working with the most vulnerable members of the public *whether or not they have a qualification*. The following categories for registration were proposed:

- **Full registration** of people with a recognised qualification
- **Transitional registration:** a temporary category covering staff in the priority groups who do not yet have a recognised qualification
- **Provisional registration:** covering new entrants to the service, with or without a recognised qualification, with conversion to full registration upon qualification.

These proposals would seem to offer protection of the most vulnerable individuals through registration of *all* care staff working with them, with or without a recognised qualification.

3.125   The improvement of quality via regulation that is proposed can be challenged on other grounds. The rate of take-up of training opportunities is slow. As we outlined earlier in this section of the report, qualification levels are low and only a small proportion of staff is currently undergoing training. This may indicate underlying problems with the approach to training. Rather than emphasising the importance of continuous professional and personal development, the acquisition of qualifications is seen by some as an end in itself, particularly through the NVQ route. NVQ has existed in social care training since 1991. Despite this, it remains unusual for new applicants to care worker positions to hold relevant qualifications. Local authorities are extremely varied in the extent to which they have encouraged take-up of NVQ training, and there has been a tendency to concentrate on using NVQs for management and administrative staff, rather than for vocational areas such as social care.[110]

3.126   The regulation of the wide range of health *support* workers is not addressed by the Care Standards Act. However, health care assistants, who undertake much of the support in nursing homes, *are* brought within it by the use of a broad definition of 'social care worker' – as a generic term encompassing the majority of people employed in social care. This is a welcome development and will end the anomalous situation, whereby someone who has been struck off as a nurse can continue to work as a health care assistant, because of the absence of any register. The regulation of health support workers more generally has still to be resolved, and proposals from the Department of Health are expected. Whatever route is chosen, it is important that it is undertaken coherently, whether this is through the United Kingdom Central Council (UKCC), or its successor, the Nurses and Midwives Council (NMC), or any other body. There is the potential to develop a joint approach with the new GSSC, and it would be a missed opportunity if this did not occur.

Training

3.127 While the emphasis on training as a core part of the strategy for improving quality of care is welcome, the Inquiry nonetheless identified a number of problems that need to be addressed, especially:

- costs of training
- variable quality of training.

The UKHCA survey of the independent sector home care workforce highlights the particular problems with training costs for smaller organisations. Indeed, they found a positive relationship between the size of organisation and likelihood of NVQ training. UKHCA quotes the comments made by a small not-for-profit organisation:

> *Some contracts do not include a training component and this puts pressure on the company to find in-house ways to train staff without incurring a cost factor.*[111]

3.128 We have already indicated the problems of tight resourcing that leaves little room for additional costs. Staff training would seem to be a major casualty of this lack of investment. The tensions between cost and quality in this area are apparent:

> *Providers of all sizes commented on the difficulties of providing training when they were faced with continued pressures from local authorities to reduce costs. The cost to the employer can be substantial ... Some local authorities did not recognise the cost of training and did not agree to pay the rates that were required by organisations with a good training programme. In some instances, local authorities turned to another organisation with lower standards, and a lower price, to provide the care.*[112]

3.129 The MEOC research on domiciliary care providers in the independent sector found a high proportion (90 per cent) of respondents stating that they paid for unqualified staff to train for qualifications. However, the researchers point out that 'it may well be that respondents did not differentiate between on-the-job induction training and qualifications'.[113] Three-quarters of the interview sample had received no help from the local authority in providing training, a factor that also emerged in submissions to the Inquiry.

3.130 Further difficulties in accessing training have been described by the Task Force on violence against social care staff, which highlighted 'structural problems' with the Training Support Programme (TSP). In effect, this reaches only the minority of social care staff employed in social services departments. Although guidance on the use of the TSP indicates that the money *can* be used to fund independent sector training, evidence to the Task Force suggested this rarely happens. This finding was supported by our Inquiry. The Task Force speculates that reasons for this situation may include:

- purchasers can only fund those agencies with whom they contract for services
- few independent sector providers have an exclusive relationship with one purchaser that might allow for this
- the money is limited and is part of funding voted for local authorities
- government advice has been that the independent sector should take responsibility for its own training and recover the costs through the fees it charges, although care providers are clear that the fees paid are not enough for them to provide the training that is needed.[114]

3.131 The Task Force concluded that the TSP mechanism is anachronistic, reflecting an era when most social care was delivered in-house, 'and cannot support targeted training priorities in the modern and diverse world of care'. Further examples of such anomalies in the funding of training were identified in the course of the Inquiry, as this comment illustrates:

> *We have no access to funding for training: we've had a go at the Treasury over this. My home is in a poor area, I have not seen a fully private patient in 22 years, but when I apply for funding they ask how many of our home residents are state funded and I say 100 per cent. They say they can't help us because that would be 'double funding'. If all your patients are private, you can get it all free!*[115]

3.132 The consequences in practice of rules that restrict use of public funds in this way appear perverse.

3.133 We were also told that the present situation contains insufficient incentives for employees to undertake training. For example, there is no established career structure in social care, and hence no clear relationship between qualification, experience or remuneration. The high turnover of staff in the care sector, which we have remarked previously, contributes to the reluctance of many employers to invest in staff, only to lose them to other (competitor) providers.

3.134 Some submissions to the Inquiry indicated employers adopting a more pragmatic approach towards training. We were told, for example:

> *You will lose some staff through training, but you keep them for the two years of training and it is likely that there will be a mutually beneficial relationship because they are going on to other things. The worst thing is to keep someone for 10 years because it is a dead end job.*[116]

3.135 The Education and Training Advisory Group of the Independent Health Care Association (IHA) told the Inquiry how training could have a positive impact. Several examples of good practice were given of training for support workers in the independent health sector. For example, BUPA have developed 'functional competencies' for health care assistants. In addition, the Elizabeth

Finn Trust (a member of the IHA), which operates residential and nursing homes throughout England, has developed a career structure to support care assistants' development. Three per cent of the budget is committed to training, and additional remuneration is provided to employees achieving NVQ levels 2 and 3. NVQ level 3 also allows the employee to move up to a new title and job description of senior care assistant, which is viewed as 'something to aspire to'. It is early days to evaluate the impact this will have on staff retention, but there was believed to be a positive effect on employees' self-esteem.[117] Other submissions have made similar observations:

> *But if you talk to those who have achieved a nationally recognised qualification for the first time in their lives, you cannot fail to be impressed. It is often a struggle against the odds, but the sense of increased self-esteem among previously downtrodden and marginalised nursing and health care assistants is inspiring.*[118]

3.136 TOPSS similarly emphasises the importance of 'Lifelong Learning' in social care, and has highlighted ways in which adults returning to education experience 'increased confidence and sense of self-achievement'.[119]

3.137 The Mental Health Foundation acknowledges that vital as training is to raising standards, it is not a panacea, and there *can* be perverse effects:

> *... this is a high risk: a new work force develops and then becomes semi-professionalised and loses its direct accountability. The issue is how you deliver a service without moving the workforce away and losing empathy with the people they support. You create an emotional distance that wasn't there before. The issue is what is the nature of the job and what do you want from people? I feel that the staff who are really good are usually those in their later working life who have made a real commitment to care, and they tend not to have huge ambitions to become managers.*[120]

Absence of a 'gold standard'

3.138   Despite the existence of the NVQ system, it is apparent that there is *not* a recognised 'gold standard'. Not all training is of equal value, and the NVQ model appears to be highly variable, particularly in inconsistent assessment, as emphasised by the following submission to the Inquiry from the Merseyside Education and Training Consortium:

> *NVQ standards vary greatly between NVQ providers despite the external verification system. There is a lack of faith in the NVQ system amongst many professional staff. This is due in part to ignorance, but also due to the lack of a clear curriculum, weakness in support of assessors and a funding arrangement for NVQs which rewards successful achievement, leading NVQ providers to be more concerned with chasing numbers than raising educational standards.*[121]

3.139   The NVQ competence-based model of training and qualification *can* work extremely well, as part of an overall approach to workforce and service management. At the heart of the approach is the use of National Occupational Standards, which combine skill, knowledge, and values. NVQs are assessed in the workplace and therefore offer the advantage of focusing on an individual's competence in their work role. Despite the strengths of the model, which should equip staff to discriminate between good and poor practice, and to challenge the latter by reference to National Occupational Standards, the NVQ system is the focus of considerable discontent. We were told for example:

> *This training is often spoon fed and of poor quality, resulting in weak standards of practice rather than the improved standard of care sought.*[122]

3.140   Some of the discontent is less about the NVQ model itself, than it is a reflection of wider workforce management deficits (such as poor supervision), which are exposed by the use of NVQ. Nonetheless, some of the criticisms *are* well founded. The quality of NVQ centres is highly variable, and a lack of standardisation has been identified as problematic by organisations seeking guarantees of support when they sign up to NVQs. The content of NVQs is also a cause of dissatisfaction, and may be inadequate in meeting the specific training needs of care workers, as this comment acknowledges:

> *We already provide a very high level of NVQ training for our staff which has proved beneficial in equipping them with some of the necessary knowledge and skills, and also acts as a motivator because it enables people to see the possibility of career progression. However, NVQ Levels 2, 3 and 4 in Care are still rather general and do not address all the specific skill requirements for working effectively with people with learning disabilities.*[123]

It is unsurprising, therefore, that many providers are seen as having 'half hearted commitment to NVQs and, at worst, no commitment at all'.[124]

National standards and training

3.141   As we have highlighted previously, the Care Standards Act (2000) seeks to drive up the quality of services through regulating staff, and by introducing new National Minimum Standards for services. These twin strategies are interlinked. The first standards have been published for care homes for older people, and standards for domiciliary care are in development; the new learning disabilities strategy also proposes an awards framework to provide relevant vocational qualifications in addition to or instead of care NVQs.[125] While many of the standards for care homes relate to the quality of the physical care environment, and the nature of daily life in the home, staffing standards are also included (see below). These have both direct and indirect implications for training, and introduce a powerful precedent for subsequent National Minimum Standards to follow. The standards are a welcome development, and we turn in Section 4 to address some of the practical implications for ensuring these standards are met and the desired outcomes realised.

Box 3.14 National standards and training requirements in care homes for older people

Standard 28

A minimum ratio of 50 per cent trained members of care staff (NVQ level two or equivalent) is achieved by 2005, excluding the registered manager and/or care manager, and in care homes providing nursing, excluding those members of the care staff who are registered nurses.

Outcome: Service users are in safe hands at all times.

Standard 30

The registered person ensures that there is a staff training and development programme which meets National Training Organisation (NTO) workforce training targets and ensures staff fulfil the aims of the home and meet the changing needs of service users.

All members of staff receive induction training to NTO specification within six weeks of appointment to their posts, including training on the principles of care, safe working practices, the organisation and worker role, the experiences and particular needs of the service user group, and the influences and particular requirements of the service setting.

All staff receive foundation training to NTO specification within the first six months of appointment, which equips them to meet the assessed needs of the service users accommodated, as defined in their individual plan of care.

All staff receive a minimum of three paid days training per year (including in-house training), and have an individual training and development assessment and profile.

Outcome: Staff are trained and competent to do their jobs.

Source: Department of Health. *Care Homes for Older People: National Minimum Standards.* London: Department of Health, 2001

Management

3.142   The final theme to emerge from our analysis of issues in the course of the Inquiry is management. This flows directly from the previous theme of regulation. Increasingly, it seemed in evidence to the Inquiry that the stress on developing robust regulatory mechanisms has been pursued at the price of overlooking many equally critical issues of *management*.

3.143   The quality of care and support is reliant on many factors, but our analysis would indicate the major importance of:

- funding
- training
- regulation
- management.

However, *management* attracts far less attention than the other components, and there are reasons to assume that the role and function of management in care and support is improperly understood or developed. The inter-relationships between these components are critical. For example, improved training and qualifications cannot be expected single-handedly to raise the quality of care. Competent and qualified staff in a poorly managed organisation will not be able to provide consistently good-quality care. There has to be a synergy between the competence of management, and of care staff.

3.144   Management incorporates a number of dimensions, including:

- supervision and control
- support
- accountability.

3.145 A consultation document on major draft National Occupational Standards for registered managers in health and social care was issued by TOPSS in February 2000. The standards were drafted to 'describe best practice in this area of work, provide an effective performance management tool to assist in workforce planning and provide a basis for the development of appropriate qualifications, training and assessment'.[126] The standards are intended for social care and nursing staff responsible for the day-to-day running of care homes. Registered managers are likely to be designated as a priority group for registration by the GSCC, and the development of the standards has been approached by TOPSS as a priority in the National Training Strategy. The Inquiry recognises the value of these standards and endorses the approach being adopted.

3.146 The National Minimum Standards for care homes have also introduced a focus on the quality of managers. It is recognised, for example, that 'the quality of care provided in a care home is strongly influenced by the calibre of the registered manager'.[127] In seeking to ensure that service users live in a care home 'which is run and managed by a person who is fit to be in charge, of good character, and able to discharge his or her responsibilities fully', Standard 31 requires the registered manager to be qualified, competent and experienced. This will include:

> *... at least 2 years experience in a senior management capacity in the managing of a relevant care setting within the past five years, and – by 2005 – has a level 4 NVQ qualification in management and care or equivalent; or if nursing care is provided, the manager is a first level registered nurse and has a relevant management qualification.*[128]

3.147 However, in contrast to these initiatives being developed for registered managers, we were struck by the generally low level of attention paid to the management and supervision of staff in both the public and independent sectors, albeit with some notable exceptions. Where there is attention to management issues in care and support, this appears to be overwhelmingly concentrated on the control of *processes* rather than on the *content and quality* of care. For example, there is a major preoccupation with time management (which is essentially about controlling costs). This is in contrast to the minimal attention given to the wider questions of good job design that plays to the strengths and interests of staff.

3.148   As we highlighted earlier, a direct result of cost containment by local authority purchasers is the reduced time spent by staff in supervision or in the office. Management of home care staff, for example, typically concentrates on directing staff to cover a given number of clients within the shortest possible time. The findings from a recent study of the home care services are striking:

> *The extent of individual supervision varied widely. Generally it seemed to be more of an aspiration than a reality. In one agency in the independent sector, it took place once every eight weeks and according to a schedule which covered client needs, procedures and other matters. In one local authority it was said never to take place at all, and in another it was virtually restricted to unusual work on child care cases. In all authorities, organisers tried to make themselves available to staff so that problems could be discussed at the latter's discretion and as they came.*

> *The main mechanisms for quality control at an individual level were complaints ... Less extreme bad practice and less extreme measures – for example, observing practice within the home – were rarely mentioned in the context of quality control ... So quality control at an individual level concentrated on rare instances when things went badly wrong rather than on raising general standards ... accurate knowledge of what was happening was limited.*[129]

3.149   The situation described above does not seem atypical to the Inquiry. Moreover, the study also suggested that managers preferred to adopt a generally hands-off approach, not least because of an awareness that they relied heavily on the goodwill of their staff.

3.150 There are grounds for assuming that management skills are under-developed both in public and in independent sector provider organisations. As Table 3.1 demonstrated earlier, management qualifications are held by low proportions of staff. Fewer than 15 per cent hold such a qualification among senior and middle rank managers in social services, while in home care services, fewer than 2 per cent hold recognised management qualifications. TOPSS UK has developed a Manager's Guide to strategic uses of National Occupational Standards. This uses the standards 'to reinforce the link from strategy to operational management and to service standards'. The guide emphasises how the standards can contribute to:

- business planning
- workforce management
- benchmarking
- change management
- contract specification for care services
- marketing
- risk management.

This is a welcome development, but there is much to be done before this strategic approach is widespread.

3.151 One reflection of poor management skills is arguably demonstrated by the lack of sophistication in commissioning and contracting processes. We have highlighted exceptions, in which commissioning is concerned with outcome specification and with detailing monitoring arrangements to ensure such outcomes are delivered. Similarly, the findings of the Joint Reviews (conducted by the Audit Commission and the Social Services Inspectorate) have highlighted the central importance of coherent management at all levels. Box 3.15 draws out some of the key messages from one such Joint Review report on the management of people delivering social services. The report emphasised that the way councils manage their employees is crucial to their ability to improve the quality of services. However, the findings suggested that:

> *... few councils have given sufficient attention to the effective management of the people they employ. Most councils could significantly improve the quality of their services, even within existing resources, by strengthening their approach to managing and supporting people, both recognising achievement and confronting unsatisfactory performance.*[130]

Box 3.15 Report of the Joint Review on the Royal Borough of Kensington and Chelsea

The report by the Joint Review Team highlighted 'impressive and intelligent frontline practice' which focuses clearly 'on the aims of intervention and outcomes for users'. The following points were made:

- Practice is underpinned by effective care management tools and exacting care management standards that are monitored by team managers.

- The management of change is supported by a forward-looking human resource strategy that places a premium upon supervision, access to training and the development of core competencies for the majority of posts.

- A key driver in securing success has been senior management's 'obsession with the frontline'.

Source: SSI/Audit Commission. A *Report of the Joint Review of Social Services in the Royal Borough of Kensington and Chelsea*. London: SSI/Audit Commission, 2001

3.152 The low recognition of the importance of management skills in care and support contrasts with the heavy emphasis placed on such development within the NHS. The NHS Plan, for example, observed that delivering the radical changes envisaged 'will require first class leaders at all levels of the NHS', and outlined proposals to deliver a step change in the calibre of NHS leadership via a new Leadership Centre for Health. We return to consider the implications of developing management skills in care and support services in Section 4 of the report.

3.153 In Section 3 of the Inquiry's report, we have highlighted our central findings across a number of key themes. These were by no means the only issues that arose in the course of the Inquiry, but they *were* the ones that were of greatest and repeated concern. Individually, many of the themes are attracting attention from a number of other quarters. However, we believe that the particular contribution of the Inquiry is to bring together these multiple issues and to emphasise their interconnections. Improving the quality of care and support demands coherent action on all these fronts, and it is to such issues that we turn in the final section.

References

[1] Department of Health. *A quality strategy for social care*. London: Stationery Office, 2000.

[2] *Ibid.*, Foreword by John Hutton, p. 3.

[3] Turner M. *It is what you do and the way that you do it: Service users views on the introduction of codes of conduct and practice for social care workers by the four national care councils*. Shaping Our Lives. National Institute for Social Work: London, 2000, p. 35.

[4] Henwood M, Lewis H, Waddington E. *Listening to users of domiciliary care services: developing and monitoring quality standards*. Leeds: Nuffield Institute for Health/United Kingdom Home Care Association, 1998, p. 5.

[5] Harding T, Beresford P. *The standards we expect: what service users and carers want from social services workers*. London: National Institute for Social Work, 1996, p. 1.

[6] Secretary of State for Health. *Modernising social services: promoting independence, improving protection, raising standards*. Cm 4169. London: The Stationery Office, 1998, para. 2.46.

[7] Commission for Racial Equality. *Race, culture and community care*. London: CRE, 1997.

[8] Patel N. Black and minority ethnic elderly: Perspectives on long term care. Chapter 9. In: *With respect to old age: long term care – rights and responsibilities: A report by the Royal Commission on Long Term Care*. Cm 4192-I. London: The Stationery Office, 1999.

[9] Department of Health, Social Care Group. *They look after their own, don't they? Inspection of community care services for black and minority ethnic minority older people*. London: Department of Health, 1998.

[10] Macpherson, Sir William. *The Stephen Lawrence Inquiry. Report of an inquiry by Sir William Macpherson of Cluny*. Cm 4262-I. London: The Stationery Office, 1999.

[11] Rose D. *Users' voices: the perspectives of mental health service users on community and hospital care*. London: The Sainsbury Centre for Mental Health, 2001, p. 94.

[12] Personal communication from Jabeer Butt, Racial Equality Unit.

[13] Audit Commission. *Charging with care: how councils charge for home care*. London: The Stationery Office, 2000, para. 14.

[14] *Ibid.*, para. 48.

[15] Mathew D, 2000. *Op. Cit.*, p. 13.

[16] Glendinning C, Halliwell S, Jacobs S, Rummery K, Tryer J. *Buying independence: using direct payments to integrate health and social services*. Bristol: The Policy Press, 2000.

[17] *Ibid.*, p. 3.

[18] *Ibid.*, p. 16.

[19] Zarb G, Nadash P. *Cashing in on independence*. Chapter 6. London: BCODP, 1994.

[20] *Ibid.*

[21] Glendinning *et al.*, 2000. *Op. Cit.*, p. 23.

[22] *Ibid.*, p. 26.

[23] 'Mind your backs' survey undertaken in 2000 by National Centre for Independent Living. *Personal assistance users news*. London: NCIL, October 2000.

[24] Zarb G, Nadash P, 1994. *Op. Cit.*

[25] Rose D, 2001. *Op. Cit.*

[26] *Ibid.*, p. 13.

[27] Biggs S, Phillipson C, Kingston P. *Elderly abuse in perspective.* Buckingham: Open University Press, 1995, p. 78.

[28] Townsend P. *The last refuge: a survey of residential institutions and homes for the aged in England and Wales.* London: Routledge and Kegan Paul, 1964.

[29] Department of Health. *Guidance on developing and implementing multi-agency policies and procedures to protect vulnerable adults from abuse.* London: The Stationery Office, 2000.

[30] Commission for Health Improvement. *Investigation into the North Lakeland NHS Trust: report to the Secretary of State for Health.* London: Commission for Health Improvement, 2000.

[31] *Ibid.*, Executive summary, para. 3.

[32] *Ibid.*, para. 21.

[33] Written submission to the Inquiry from the Royal College of Physicians.

[34] Jenkins G, Asif Z, Bennett G. *Listening is not enough – an analysis of calls to elder abuse.* London: Action on Elder Abuse, 2000.

[35] *Ibid.*, p. 17.

[36] Mathew D. *Who cares? A profile of the independent sector home care workforce in England.* Carshalton Beeches: UKHCA, 2000.

[37] Health Committee. *Third report. Community care: funding from April 1992*, 309–1. London: HMSO, para. 71.

[38] Audit Commission. *Taking care: progress with care in the community.* Bulletin No.1. London: Audit Commission, 1993.

[39] UNISON, written submission to the Inquiry.

[40] Gowland D, Taylor M. *A good job in care? A practical approach to localising the equalities agenda for improvements to employment in health and social care.* Harlow: South & East Economic Development Strategy, 1999

[41] Wistow G, Knapp M, Hardy B, Allen C. *Social care in a mixed economy.* Buckingham: Open University Press, 1994.

[42] Wistow G, Knapp M, Hardy B, Forder J, Kendall J, Manning R. *Social care markets: progress and prospects.* Buckingham: Open University Press, 1996.

[43] Knapp M, Hardy B, Forder J. Commissioning for quality: ten years of social care markets in England. *Journal of Social Policy* 2001; 30: 2.

[44] Knapp M, Forder J, Kendall J, Pickard L. The growth of independent sector provision in the UK. In: Harper S, editors. *The family in an ageing society.* Oxford: Oxford University Press, 2001 (in press).

[45] *Ibid.*

[46] Browning D. *With respect to old age: long term care – rights and responsibilities. A report of the Royal Commission on Long Term Care.* Research Volume 3. Chapter 8 'Value for Money'. Cm 4192-II/3. London: The Stationery Office, 1999, p. 117.

[47] Capital Carers, written submission to the Inquiry.

[48] Matosevic T, Knapp M, Kendall J, Forder J, Ware P, Hardy B. *Domiciliary care providers in the independent sector.* PSSRU Monograph. LSE: London, 2001.

[49] Bill McClimont, UKHCA, oral evidence to the Inquiry, 18 September 2000.

[50] Matosevic *et al.*, 2001. *Op. Cit.*

[51] Care assistant, written submission to the Inquiry.

[52] Rickford F. Value judgements. *Community Care* 2000: 16–22 November, pp. 21–22.

[53] Knapp M, Hardy B, Forder J, 2001. *Op. Cit.*

[54] *Ibid.*

[55] Secretary of State for Health. *Modernising social services.* Cm 4169. London: The Stationery Office, 1998.

[56] Audit Commission. *Another step forward.* London: Audit Commission, 2001.

[57] Department of Health, Social Care Group. *That's the way the money goes: inspection of commissioning arrangements for Community Care Services.* London: Department of Health, 1999.

[58] *Ibid.,* para. 1.5.

[59] *Ibid.,* para. 4.3.

[60] *Ibid.,* para. 4.20.

[61] *Ibid.,* para. 4.28.

[62] Gowland D, Taylor M, 1999. *Op. Cit.,* p. 48.

[63] Secretary of State for Health, 1998. *Op. Cit.,* p. 37

[64] Department of Health. *Modern social services. A commitment to people.* The ninth annual report of the Chief Inspector of Social Services. London: Department of Health, 2000, para 1.16.

[65] John Belcher, Anchor Trust, oral evidence to the Inquiry, 18 September 2000.

[66] Merseyside Education and Training Consortium, written submission to the Inquiry.

[67] Training Standards Council. *Training in care.* London: Training Standards Council, 2000, p. 5.

[68] Sutherland S. *With respect to old age: long term care - rights and responsibilities. A report of the Royal Commission on Long Term Care.* London: The Stationery Office, 1999.

[69] Mathew D, 2000. *Op. Cit.*

[70] Royal National Institute for the Deaf, written submission to the Inquiry.

[71] Stroke Association, written submission to the Inquiry.

[72] Alcohol Problems Advisory Service, written submission to the Inquiry.

[73] Independent consultant John Hudson, written submission to the Inquiry.

[74] Turner M, 2000. *Op. Cit.,* p. 20.

[75] Turner M, 2000. *Op. Cit.,* p. 12.

[76] TOPSS England. *Modernising the social care workforce - the first national training strategy for England.* London: TOPSS, 2000, para. 2.2.

[77] Association for Residential Care, written submission to the Inquiry.

[78] Matosevic *et al.,* 2001. *Op. Cit.,* p. 18

[79] Audit Commission/SSI. *People need people: releasing the potential of people working in social services.* London: Audit Commission, 2000.

[80] *Ibid.,* p. 17.

[81] Gowland D, Taylor M, 1999. *Op. Cit*

[82] Gowland D, Taylor M, 1999. *Op. Cit.,* p.82

[83] Taylor M. *Home care: the forgotten service. Report on UNISON's survey of home care workers in the UK.* London: UNISON, 2001.

[84] *Op. Cit.*

[85] UNISON, written submission to the Inquiry.

[86] TOPSS England, 2000. *Op. Cit.,* para. 2.3.6.

[87] Platt D. The challenges which face the social services workforce. Speech to Guardian/NISW Conference, London, 3 November, 2000.

[88] Hunter M. Recruitment crisis looms for home care. *Community Care* 1999; 19–25 August, 1999, pp. 8–9

[89] Matosevic *et al,* 2001. *Op. Cit.*, p. 20.

[90] Raymond A. Everyone a winner. *Community Care* 1999; 12–18 April, p. 23.

[91] Julia Twigg, University of Kent, oral evidence to the Inquiry, 18 September, 2000.

[92] Twigg J. *Bathing – the body and community care.* Andover: Taylor and Francis Group, 2000, p. 124.

[93] *Ibid.*

[94] National Task Force on Violence Against Social Care Staff. *A safer place: report and national action plan.* London: Department of Health, 2001.

[95] National Task Force on Violence against Social Care Staff. *Report on qualitative research among social care organisations.* London: Department of Health, 2000, p. 1.

[96] Research Perspectives. *Violence against social care staff.* London: Research Perspectives, 2000, p. 2.

[97] National Task Force on Violence against Social Care Staff, 2001. *Op. Cit.*, para. 5.1.

[98] National Task Force on Violence against Social Care Staff, 2000. *Op. Cit.*, p. 1

[99] *Ibid.*, para. 10.3

[100] Henwood, Lewis, Waddington, 1998. *Op. Cit.*, p. 8.

[101] UNISON. *Racial harassment? It's not part of the job! UNISON guidelines for handling racial harassment by patients and service users.* London: UNISON, 1996.

[102] Research Perspectives, 2000. *Op. Cit.*, p. 26.

[103] Secretary of State for Health, 1998. *Op. Cit.*, para. 5.6.

[104] Secretary of State for Health, 1998. *Op. Cit.*, para. 5.7.

[105] Brand D, Smith G. *Social care registration project: Consultation paper on proposals for a draft registration scheme for the social care workforce.* London: NISW & OLM Consulting, 2001.

[106] Care Standards Act 2000. *Explanatory notes.* London: The Stationery Office, 2000, para. 154.

[107] UNISON, written submission to the Inquiry.

[108] National Institute for Social Work. *The need for a general social services council.* London: NISW, 1992, para. 11.

[109] *Ibid.*, para. 11.

[110] Platt S. Qualifying rounds. *Community Care* 1997; 30 January, pp. 32–3.

[111] Mathew D, 2000. *Op. Cit.*, p. 28

[112] *Ibid.*, p. 29.

[113] Matosevic *et al.*, 2001. *Op. Cit.*, p. 18

[114] National Task Force on Violence Against Social Care Staff, 2001. *Op. Cit.*, para. 8.3.

[115] British Federation of Care Home Proprietors, oral evidence to the Inquiry, 18 September, 2000.

[116] Ginny Jenkins, Action on Elder Abuse, oral evidence to the Inquiry, 23 October, 2000.

[117] Independent Healthcare Association, oral evidence to the Inquiry, 23 October, 2000.

[118] Chapman P. A snapshot in time. *Nursing Times* 1997; 93: pp. 26–28.

[119] TOPSS UK. *Experiences in lifelong learning.* London: TOPSS.

[120] Mental Health Foundation, oral evidence to the Inquiry, 23 October, 2000.

[121] Merseyside Education and Training Consortium, written submission to the Inquiry.

[122] First Community Health NHS Trust, written submission to the Inquiry.

[123] Surrey Oaklands NHS Trust, written submission to the Inquiry.

[124] Hoskins C. NVQs: it's time they got the recognition they deserve. *Nursing Times Learning Curve* 1999; 3 (7).

[125] Department of Health. *Valuing people: a new strategy for learning disability for the 21st century.* London: The Stationery Office, 2001.

[126] TOPSS England. *Consultation on draft national occupational standards for registered managers in health and social care.* London: TOPSS, 2000.

[127] Department of Health. *Care homes for older people: national minimum standards.* London: The Stationery Office, 2001, p. 37

[128] *Ibid.,* Standard 31.

[129] Sinclair I, Gibbs I, Hicks L. *The management and effectiveness of the home care service.* (Draft report.) York: University of York, 2000, p. 32.

[130] Audit Commission, 2000. *Op. Cit.,* p. 3.

4   Conclusions and recommendations

4.1   Section 3 presented our analysis of the key themes that arose in the course of the Inquiry. Although we recognise that many issues are involved, we have concentrated on those themes that arose as the most significant factors in terms of: cost and quality; skills and values; staffing; regulation and training; and management. In this final section, we draw together the main conclusions from the analysis and present our recommendations for the way forward.

Quality

Investment

> *It is apparent that the quality of care and support services falls far short of what users and carers should be able to expect. While a minority of services may be of a really poor standard, many are mediocre.*

4.2   We recognise that the quality of social care and support is considerably better in many ways than in the past, and that the community care reforms, for example, have had a considerable impact. However, quality continues to fall short of what should be a reasonable expectation. Despite increasing recognition of the shortcomings that exist, the changes being put in place to raise quality are, in themselves, unlikely to be sufficient. While many factors need to be addressed in raising quality, the starting point has to be the adequacy of overall investment. The conclusion is inescapable that the social care sector is significantly under-resourced.

> *There is gross under-investment in social care and support, and significant additional resources are required.*

4.3   We are struck by the contrast between the situation in social care, and that which is emerging in the health service. The NHS Plan has clearly recognised the consequences of decades of under-investment in health services, and the Government has pledged to inject major real investment year-on-year in order to raise standards and make up for past shortfalls. We are convinced of the necessity for similar major investment in the care and support services. The scale of investment required is uncertain. This is partly because care and support services are provided in an environment characterised by change and unpredictability, with major changes occurring in demography, socio-economic factors and availability of informal care, and with many layers of direct and indirect variables. We are also limited in our analysis by the data available. However, the PSSRU long-term care financing model for older people indicates the following:

- Merely to stand still and maintain services for older people at current levels will require an increase in public finance from £6.8 billion in 2000 to £8.1 billion by 2010 and £10.5 billion by 2020.

- If services were to be provided in a 'carer-blind' approach, i.e. without taking into account whether or not service users had informal carers, there would need to be an 80 per cent increase in the level of home care services needed between 2000 and 2031. This should be compared to an increase of just under 50 per cent on the base case.

4.4   The capacity of the Department of Health to deliver its modernisation agenda in health and social care will be seriously compromised without attention to these matters. The pressures on services to deliver within tighter and tighter financial constraints has had direct effects on the nature of the care and support provided. Support is increasingly reduced to a series of tasks and interventions, rather than the provision of supportive, flexible and responsive, individualised care. Not only is this precisely the opposite of what service users want, but it also makes it virtually impossible to pursue the vital policy objectives of maximising independence and preventing physical and psychological decline.

> ### *Recommendation 1*
>
> We urge the Government to recognise the significant under-investment in care and support services, and to commit itself to making good the substantial shortfalls that have occurred year-on-year. We believe that the order of investment required is likely to be at least the same as that being injected into the NHS, i.e. a growth of approximately half in cash terms, and one-third in real terms in just five years. Without such investment, care and support services will be struggling to stand still. They will be unable to address the major improvements needed in quality or to meet the additional requirements of new national standards.

Choice and control

Many service users fail to experience any significant choice or control over the services that they receive.

4.5   Particular concerns arise over the lack of choice and control that most services users experience. Although there is a lot of rhetoric around the concepts of user empowerment and involvement, a considerable gap exists between rhetoric and reality. There are good examples of the successful use of Direct Payments, which place power with service users and enable them to buy in and organise their own services. However, the limited uptake of such schemes points both to their likely limitations and probably inadequate support and promotion of the schemes by individual local authorities. Direct Payments will not be the answer for everyone, and it is important to try and incorporate the valued features of the Direct Payment model into mainstream care and support. It is possible for service users to exercise meaningful choices and experience greater control, when individual care planning is implemented properly.

Recommendation 2

The continued development of Direct Payments must be actively promoted. This demands a more proactive approach by the Department of Health, and by local authorities and Care Trusts, in encouraging and supporting take-up of services. This includes giving service users the training and skills they need to become their own service commissioners and care managers. For those service users who do not want to, or are unable, to make use of Direct Payments, other ways (e.g. care planning) must be found of ensuring that real choices and control are built into the use of care and support services. These are vital factors that drive forward service quality.

Services that are culturally responsive to the diversity of needs of people in black and minority ethnic communities are poorly developed, despite some notable examples of success.

4.6   Service users from black and minority ethnic communities may experience even less choice or control over services because of the poor accessibility and responsiveness of services. There are many examples of successful developments, both in local authority services and in specialist services, the latter often developed by black and minority ethnic voluntary groups. Improving services requires a twin approach that promotes local grass-roots solutions while also emphasising the need to address responsiveness within mainstream services.

Recommendation 3

Commissioners of care and support services must encourage the development of a wide range of services to meet the diverse needs of different communities. However, addressing these needs is not something which can be left to specialist services. A key test of mainstream services must be the extent to which they respond appropriately to service users from all cultural and racial backgrounds. We recommend that the Department of Health pays proper attention to addressing racial equalities issues within the emerging National Minimum Standards agenda. Disseminating information about successful examples of innovative services should be an important early responsibility of the new Social Care Institute for Excellence.

User involvement and empowerment are words that are in frequent use, but often with little consideration of what they mean in practice, either at the level of the individual, or collectively.

4.7   Moving beyond rhetoric and tokenism, it is striking that innovative approaches to user involvement in quality monitoring have enormous potential. Examples, such as the User-Focused Monitoring (UFM) of mental health services, from the Sainsbury Centre for Mental Health, point to the scope for participation by people who are frail or who have considerable incapacity. Not only does UFM offer a route into monitoring services in which the reality of service quality is more likely to be exposed, but the experience is extremely positive for those taking part. 'offer a route into services in which the reality of service quality is more likely to be exposed'.

4.8   The development of similar approaches to training should be encouraged. The direct involvement of service users is invaluable in raising awareness and understanding of the needs of service users. It also ensures staff training is better related to those needs.

> **Recommendation 4**
>
> We strongly endorse the genuine involvement and empowerment of service users. Users have a vital role to play in areas such as service monitoring and review, and in training staff to better understand users' needs and the principles which should inform care and support. We urge both the Commission for Health Improvement and the Social Care Institute for Excellence to identify the characteristics of successful examples of such practices and to encourage their widespread adoption.

Cost and quality tensions

Care staff provide a highly valued and essential service for millions of people, and the commitment and dedication of many staff cannot be faulted.

4.9   The pressures on care and support staff are enormous. Many provide an excellent service, often far above and beyond that which might be expected. However, there are grounds for believing that, without radical change, there is potential for a major deterioration in standards of care.

Major expenditure constraints that have forced local authorities to systematically drive down costs are now biting into the quality of services that can be provided.

4.10   The conclusion is unmistakable that the requirement to bear down on costs has led to a damaging preoccupation with price at the expense of quality. We accept that the concept of Best Value is intended to address both cost and quality issues. However, the evidence to the Inquiry demonstrated repeatedly that cost control has left virtually no room for further efficiencies. In some instances, the impact on service quality is threatening the continuation of the social care market. There is a point at which the parallel objectives of securing continuous improvements in service quality, while also making efficiency savings, generate conflicting tensions.

Recommendation 5

We are concerned that the tool of 'Best Value' risks being discredited by the disproportionate emphasis which, in practice, is being laid on driving down costs, at the price of quality. We urge the DETR, the Audit Commission and the National Care Standards Commission to review guidance on Best Value to ensure there is adequate recognition that improving service quality is not always synonymous with driving down contract prices.

Commissioning for quality

Large-scale service provider companies are usually the best placed to survive the pressures of the market place, while smaller companies are exposed to greater proportionate risks. Although we would not argue that small is necessarily best, questions do need to be asked about whether the market is managed in ways that have sufficient regard to its complexities.

Commissioning of care and support services is relatively unsophisticated. Progress is evident in moving from adversarial style relationships to greater co-operation, but this requires considerable development.

4.11   Most commissioning and contracting of care and support services (whether 'in house' or in the independent sector) is unsophisticated: it is poorly related to outcomes and pays little regard to levers that might raise service quality. This may partly be due to the relative immaturity of the market. However, it is also likely to be related to poor development of management skills within local authorities. The relationships between purchasers and providers are rarely characterised by partnership, or a genuine understanding. Commissioners seem to have little sense of which aspects of commissioning and contracting need to be kept 'tight', and which should be 'loose'. This can create restrictive contracts that allow little, or no scope, for flexibility or response to changing needs. There is an urgent need to develop commissioning and to move away from a largely bureaucratic and controlling approach, to the creative promotion of desired outcomes, balanced by appropriate checks and quality assurance processes.

Recommendation 6

There is an urgent need to develop commissioning capacity and skills. We propose the Department of Health should issue new guidance to local authorities, Primary Care Trusts and Care Trusts, on best practice in commissioning. This guidance should focus on how best to promote the development of high quality, creative and responsive services. This needs to be matched by strategies to develop and support commissioning capacity and skills, and there is a clear agenda for the training requirements for commissioning managers.

The changing structures in health and social care have profound implications for future service commissioning – particularly concerning the emergence of new Care Trusts.

4.12 The NHS Plan signalled major changes to the relationships between health and local authorities, with a move away from the old models of collaboration and co-operation and towards a form of integration. These developments have considerable potential to increase the coherence of services, and to overcome 'the old divisions' between health and social care. Although there are opportunities for improving the health and care response to complex needs through Care Trusts, there are also risks in rushing ahead with an untested and insufficiently developed model, and in allowing implementation to lead policy rather than the reverse. The 'emerging framework' that has been issued by the

Department of Health acknowledges that 'the policy is being developed as the detailed issues emerge and are considered'.[1] Positive outcomes may result. However, this incremental approach is not underpinned by a coherent policy or evidence base. Moreover, in basing the Care Trusts on existing Primary Care Trusts there are particular concerns about the implications of the health service assuming a commissioning role in which it has little experience.

Recommendation 7

The development of Care Trusts must be approached with caution, rather than 'driven through' as an ideological objective. There are many aspects of the commissioning role in these Trusts that need to be better developed. The Department of Health must take responsibility for appropriate governance arrangements. It must also ensure there is an appropriate level of understanding and knowledge about the needs of service users, by ensuring parity of health and social care interests.

Training and qualifications

Reviewing NVQ

The Care NVQ system is the focus of considerable discontent. In view of the very strong emphasis being attached to attainment of NVQ by national standards, a major review and overhaul of assessment and verification of NVQ is required.

4.13 We conclude that the shortcomings of Care NVQs demand the urgent attention of the Qualifications and Curriculum Authority (QCA), and awarding bodies, to tackle the problems of consistency of assessment. Increasingly, training staff to a recognised standard will no longer be an option, but a requirement. It is essential that this requirement is meaningful and offers a gold standard. The attainment of a Care NVQ has to be something that is seen as a sound and reliable indicator of a competent worker.

Recommendation 8

We recommend three complementary actions to address shortcomings with NVQs:

- The QCA, and awarding bodies offering Care NVQs, should undertake an immediate review to determine the consistency of assessment, and take any necessary action arising.
- A review of the National Occupational Standards that provide the content of Care NVQs is underway by TOPSS and Healthwork UK, and due to be completed by 2003. We recommend that as part of the review, work should be undertaken to strengthen assessment requirements and improve consistency.
- Work should be undertaken by TOPSS and Healthwork UK to improve the quality of work-based assessment through better support to line managers undertaking assessment.

Skills and competence

We recognise the vital contribution of continuous development of staff and recognition of the value of experience.

4.14   We accept that there are strong associations between poor practices and poor training. The care and support sector suffers from a history and tradition of employing unqualified labour. Despite major changes in the nature of the work, and increasing demands on staff to provide better and more responsive services to people with a growing range of complex needs, the image remains one of low skill work that 'anyone can do'.

4.15   Care and support staff bring a wealth of experience that workforce management systems, including training, need to recognise and build upon. Training must ensure that staff develop their skills and knowledge, but many training approaches are focused principally on the development of technical competence. While we accept that these skills are needed, it is equally clear that such training is of little use, unless it is accompanied by the awareness and application of certain core values. These include, for example, principles of: individuality, identity, rights, choice, privacy, independence, dignity, respect and partnership, equal opportunities and confidentiality, such as underpin the TOPPS induction standards. The 'poor attitudes' that have been identified by services users in a minority of support workers are indicative of the failure of care providers to promote and reinforce basic principles of care.

Recommendation 9

We recommend that TOPSS and Healthwork UK urgently progress work to ensure that all training builds on the skills of staff and develops competence on the basis of appropriate qualifications. Equal weight must be given to developing underlying values and attitudes, as to the acquisition of practical and technical skills. The identification of appropriate learning routes to qualifications should be a priority.

Supporting the costs of training

The costs to independent providers of investing in training are a significant disincentive to provide employees with more than the basic minimum induction.

4.16   The costs of training staff can be significant, and particularly in a situation of high staff turnover, employers do not have the incentives to invest in training. With qualification and training requirements increasingly mandatory, questions remain about how the take-up of training can best be supported across both the public and independent sectors. This is likely to require a number of complementary strategies. Although the Department of Health recognises that 'the need to raise qualification levels in the voluntary and independent sectors is as much a part of the Government's plans as in the statutory sector,'[2] providers often reported difficulties to the Inquiry in obtaining access to training, or in recouping the costs involved. It is vital that local authorities work with providers to address training requirements.

4.17   We recognise that other strategies may also be required. For example, the announcement in the NHS Plan of 'Individual Learning Accounts' (ILAs) for NHS staff who do not have a professional qualification, is an innovative model that could be adapted for application to care and support. In fact, ILAs have been established as part of the Government's Lifelong Learning strategy, aimed at raising the skills of the workforce. They are available to anyone aged over 19. They provide a financial incentive and discounts on training courses leading to a recognised qualification (currently up to £150, or £200 for information technology, in any single year). There is considerable scope for building on the ILAs, and enhancing their value through third party contributions. More broadly, the establishment of the Learning and Skills Council offers a further opportunity to experiment with different approaches to enhancing training and raising skills.

Recommendation 10

Local authorities must work with providers to raise the skills and standards of all care staff. Supporting the costs of training staff to higher standards necessitates that providers are able to reflect the realistic costs of training within their contract prices, and/or that local authorities ensure access to the resources of the Training Support Programme. We also recommend that TOPSS, Healthwork UK and the new Learning and Skills Council should consider financial incentives for employers and employees to train and achieve higher level skills by means of:

- ILAs enhanced through additional contributions from employers and/or regulators
- training loans – including transferable training loans – targeted especially at independent sector providers.

We recommend the piloting of these models as a matter of urgency.

Staffing – the heart of health and care

Recruitment and retention

Recruitment and retention of staff in care and support services represents a major – and growing – challenge that demands a range of imaginative and creative response if crisis is to be avoided.

4.18   There is enormous uncertainty surrounding the future supply of care in both the formal (public, private and voluntary) and informal sectors. It is essential in such conditions to take all possible steps to encourage people to enter the care sector. However, at the very time when there is a growing need for care, there are powerful combinations of factors militating against attracting personnel. There are also tensions between the desire to raise standards in services and the need to avoid introducing additional barriers to entry for prospective employees.

4.19   There are substantial problems with recruitment and retention of the caring labour force. Similar problems exist in other key areas of the service sector, especially nursing and teaching, and there is growing competition for a dwindling pool of labour. It is imperative that workforce planning is undertaken collaboratively between health and social care. We welcome the opportunity provided by the new NHS Workforce Confederations, and by the Regional Training Forums established by TOPSS, both of which could facilitate a partnership approach.[3]

4.20   The greatest competitors for care and support workers are other areas of low-paid and low-skilled work, particularly in the retail sector. We have already emphasised the need for major investment in care and support, part of which should be directed towards raising the image and status of the work. The low status, which is currently reflected in poor pay and conditions of employment, does not help recruit potential employees from new sources, and a radical change in status is needed.

4.21   Unlike the nursing and teaching professions, in which financial and other incentives are increasingly considered necessary to attract and retain high-quality staff, there has been virtually no debate of similar issues for care and support workers. This reinforces the low status of the sector, and the view that it is non-professional work that 'anyone can do'. We believe that changing the perceived status of the sector is of fundamental importance. This also requires a shift in attitudes towards the people being cared for by health and care services. The low status of much care work may partly reflect the low status that society attaches to elderly and disabled people. Changing such attitudes takes time. However, we welcome, for example, the National Service Framework for Older People which, for the first time, tackles discrimination in health and care services on the basis of age.

4.22   Recent media interest in raising the profile of care has been welcome, and potentially influential. A highly praised series of features in The Guardian on 'The Common Good' in early 2001 underlined the valued work undertaken by public servants. The joint campaign to raise awareness of the value of social workers, established by Community Care magazine and the Local Government Association has been similarly well received and has attracted government support. We welcome the pledge by John Hutton MP that the Department of Health will pursue strategies to raise the profile of social work and social care and boost recruitment. This is to be built around a series of local initiatives targeted at areas with the most serious problems. What those initiatives might look like remains to be seen, and we offer our own recommendations below.

Recommendation 11

We urge the Department of Health to be imaginative and flexible in developing strategies to raise the status and image of the care and support sector, and to recognise that these must go far beyond reforming social work training. At the heart of this must be realistic and appropriate remuneration for highly demanding work, improved conditions of employment and career prospects. Other approaches to enhancing the status of care workers should be piloted, including exploring the effects of different titles (such as 'personal care assistants', or 'community care workers') that better reflect the skilled and valued work which care workers undertake. Other experimentation with changing the pattern of incentives might focus on extending 'key worker' status to care and support workers in localities where there are particular problems with recruitment and retention.

The Department of Health should give the lead in promoting strategies to improve recruitment and retention, and successful approaches in both the health and care sectors should be widely shared.

4.23   Improving recruitment and retention must be the responsibility of a number of different stakeholders. In addition to the central lead that needs to be given by the Department of Health, service purchasers and providers also have a vital role to play. We are aware that care providers are already pursuing a range of approaches to addressing the challenges of staff recruitment and retention. From the Inquiry, we are convinced that some innovative approaches are worth developing more widely, and it is essential that successful experiences are shared. Of particular interest are approaches seeking to attract a richer mix of varied staff, including those who may not fit the conventional model of care worker. Strategies are needed that focus on attracting both the young and the more mature. For example, there is the opportunity presented by the proposed development of vocationally related GCSEs. In contrast, at the other end of the working life, it may be possible to attract staff who have left the labour market in their 50s, or who are newly retired. Some of these people will welcome part-time and flexible work, and will bring a range of skills from a lifetime of experience, not necessarily spent in the care or nursing sectors.

4.24   While we have emphasised the benefits of continuity of care and opportunities to build relationships between service users and care staff, we also recognise there is a contribution to be made by people who only intend to remain in care work for a relatively short time. The recruitment of a more transient group of workers (such as young people working in a 'gap year', or people on their way to other careers via care work), as one component of a flexible labour force, could be an important part of an innovative workforce strategy.

4.25   The experience of some providers has also underlined the benefits of developing and supporting particular communities of interest (e.g. of faith, culture or locality). People are motivated by different considerations – some may not be attracted in general by the idea of care work, but may be interested if the work helped support a community about which they cared and identified with. We have seen successful examples of this approach both in support for particular groups of service users (e.g. people with mental health needs, or people with HIV/AIDs), and for different minority ethnic groups, where the concept of the 'interdependency' of people can be especially powerful in motivating support. There is scope for extending this approach to a wide range of different types of 'community' in both urban and rural settings.

Recommendation 12

We recommend that the remit of the National Workforce Development Board in the Department of Health should be a wide one that goes beyond health care. This would provide a particular opportunity to address the interdependencies between the health and care employment sectors. The Development Board should take responsibility for identifying and disseminating examples of successful recruitment and retention strategies in health and care that might be more widely adopted.

The contribution of volunteers

The contribution of volunteers can make an important difference to service users' experiences and satisfactions. A complementary role for volunteers needs to be supported and encouraged. However, this is not a substitute for adequate staffing, and must not be viewed as a cheap option.

4.26   There has always been – and will continue to be – an important role for volunteers in many areas of care. As we have already remarked, the changing demography of the developed world is re-casting the nature of mid-life and early old age, and there are many people in their 50s and 60s who have retired, or partially retired, from work, but who remain fit and active. Many of these people might be attracted into part-time paid care work, but there is also scope for encouraging voluntary activity, with government policy supporting the expansion of voluntary activity at all stages of the life cycle. However, although there are opportunities for volunteers to make a further contribution to health and care, this is by no means a ready solution to the problems of labour supply, or an easy substitute for a skilled and trained workforce.

4.27   We are concerned that without careful planning in the care and support field, an overemphasis on using volunteers could in fact be counterproductive. It is usually easier to attract volunteers to the more satisfying aspects of care giving, such as befriending and visiting. However, there is the danger that separating out the more attractive elements of care will further fragment the nature of care work, leaving the most demanding and difficult work for paid carers. In addition, the problems of staff retention also affect volunteers, many of whom do not want to continue to volunteer in the long term.

4.28   The safeguards that need to be built in to any volunteer programme can be a disincentive to smaller voluntary organisations, for whom the costs of police check procedures can be onerous, and may encourage the avoidance of proper vetting processes. From the autumn of 2001, with the establishment of the

Criminal Records Bureau, there will be new procedures responsible for providing a 'one-stop' disclosure service. There has been a positive response to pressure from the voluntary sector to waive the disclosure fee for volunteers working with children and vulnerable adults.

Recommendation 13

Measures to encourage volunteering in health and care need to understand the complementary role which volunteers play, and not treat them as substitute labour. The Government's enthusiasm for volunteers, and its emphasis on the responsibilities of everyone in a civic society must be matched by the development of a Charter for volunteers that addresses their rights, as well as those of the people they support. The need for adequate quality safeguards to check the suitability of volunteers is vital and the operation of the new Criminal Records Bureau will need to be carefully monitored to ensure that it is meeting disclosure requirements.

Intelligent regulation

> *The Care Standards Act (2000) has introduced new structures and regulatory mechanisms that have enormous potential to transform the shape of social care. However, delivering this agenda is a major challenge that needs to overcome many hurdles, including the complexity of multiple new structures and layers of different regulatory bodies. The need is to develop approaches that are 'intelligent' in style and avoid the pitfalls of heavily resourced bureaucracies.*

4.29   The Government's approach to securing wholesale improvements in care and support is based around the introduction of a new system of regulation and development of new National Minimum Standards. This is a welcome recognition of the shortcomings in existing regulatory arrangements. However, we are concerned that a focus on registration, and on qualification as the sole path to registration, is misplaced because of the considerable delay this will cause before the aspirations of the Care Standards Act can be delivered. Furthermore, by default, there will be an interim period during the early years of registration in which a two-tier system will operate.

4.30   If the registration of care and support workers is seen as the key to the protection of service users, we are deeply concerned about the resulting considerable period of delay before this objective can be attained. The idea that it is acceptable to delay registration of a group of care workers until the level of qualification has reached a critical mass is fundamentally flawed. The Inquiry recognises that a two-tier system is far from ideal, and could suggest a return to the difficulties that existed, for example, with 'registered' and 'enrolled' nurses. However, we believe that, by default, there will be such a system as an interim stage – a situation that must be addressed. The present plans for registration via qualification tackle only one dimension, and it is essential that the much larger group of unqualified staff are also brought within the remit of registration.

Recommendation 14

We recommend that the General Social Care Council should adopt a revised timetable for the registration of care workers that does not rely solely on registration based on qualification. An interim register should also be developed that includes all unqualified social care workers employed by local authorities and in the independent sector, and establishes target dates for their full registration on the basis of qualification. We also urge that in bringing forward proposals for the regulation of health support workers, the Department of Health is mindful of the opportunity for – and importance of – developing a coherent approach between the remit of the General Social Care Council and whatever additional regulatory body is given responsibility in the health field.

4.31   Regulation can be a blunt instrument, and we urge adoption of an 'intelligent' approach fit for its purpose. Imposing rules without any flexibility of interpretation is unhelpful. Examples of rules that can impede the delivery of appropriate service include health and safety regulations. Although we accept the need for protection of both care workers and service users, it is equally clear that there needs to be some latitude in the way in which such rules are interpreted. We welcome the development of National Minimum Standards in services because they will enable service users to know what they should expect in their care, and provide a benchmark against which services can be held to account. We recognise that these standards need to be seen as evolutionary rather than fixed in stone, and that they will need to develop to reflect changing expectations. Standards must not be set at such low levels that their achievement is meaningless, but neither must they be set so high that they are unrealistic and have a major deleterious impact on the ability of many good services to continue operating.

Management development

Management infrastructure and capacity in social care has been one of the key casualties of financial restraint, and without significant development of leadership and management skills at all levels to provide a coherent management chain throughout the organisation, the capacity to deliver quality services will be seriously compromised.

4.32   Finally, we are struck by the need to address management issues. We do not believe that investment in the care sector will, in itself, succeed in fundamentally raising quality unless attention is paid at the same time to how the money is used and for what results.

4.33   Management capacity is under-developed in social care, and relatively little attention has been paid to addressing this. We do not believe it is possible to achieve the step change required in the quality of care and support services without serious attention to the development of management skills. Although we welcome, for example, the moves to address standards for registered managers in residential care, this is just one part of a much wider strategy that needs urgent development.

4.34   Workforce planning is an important part of management. As the findings from the Joint Review have underlined, 'councils that are performing best in service delivery and the management of performance and resources, are also those that score highly on their management of staff. Those that are performing poorly overall usually need to improve their management of people.'[4] The emphasis on raising quality and meeting new national standards in health and care demands improvements in management at all levels. The NHS Plan emphasised the need for clinical and managerial leaders throughout the health service. It acknowledged the need for change from the ad hoc and incoherent approach to leadership development within the health service. The same observations are even more applicable to the social care arena. While some improvements have been put in place (e.g. the Top Managers Programme), a more comprehensive strategy is now required.

4.35   As the Chief Inspector of Social Services acknowledged in the 2000 Annual Report, 'organisations support quality in their staff by ensuring their development, providing proper management supervision and appraisal and quality assurance systems to support competent practice.'[5] Further means of achieving these developments are needed, and innovative approaches should be encouraged.

Recommendation 15

There is an undeniable need to invest in the development of management and leadership skills across the public and independent sectors of care and support. We recommend the urgent development of appropriate management training as a priority. The Department of Health should take the lead in supporting management development at all organisational levels. Requirements to obtain management qualifications and skills must be matched by opportunities to do so, and there may be scope for building on the foundation of Individual Learning Accounts to encourage take-up by employees and employers alike.

4.36   Failure to tackle this demanding agenda would be short-sighted, and for the millions of current and future service users and their carers, it could indeed be catastrophic. The future will always be imperfect, but we believe that the solutions we are offering have the potential to transform the quality of care and support services.

References

[1] Department of Health. *Care Trusts: emerging framework.* London: Department of Health, 2001.

[2] Department of Health. *Information pack for the 2001/2002 training support programme circular LAC (2001)7.* London: Department of Health, 2001.

[3] *Ibid.*

[4] *Ibid.*, para. 18.

[5] Social Service Inspectorate. *Modern social services: a commitment to people. The ninth annual report of the Chief Inspector of Social Services 1999/2000.* London: Department of Health, 2000, para. 1.17.

Appendix 1

The social care workforce and services

Adelina Comas-Herrera, Tihana Matosevic and Jeremy Kendall[1]

This appendix presents a profile of the social care workforce (numbers of staff employed in social care, their age, gender, ethnicity and their qualifications and training); expenditure on different services; and the proportion of public expenditure costs that are recovered through charges. It also includes some evidence about the wage levels paid to care and support workers, terms and conditions of employment, and staff turnover.

During the process of this review, a number of limitations with the evidence base became clear. Specialised studies in the area of the social care workforce and services have been small in scale, examining the workforce issues for a small number of client groups, and localised to particular areas of the country. Information on the social care staff and services are more readily identifiable for older people than for other client groups. Other limitations of the information about the social care workforce are:

- for some services (e.g. sheltered housing) the data was difficult to find
- information on publicly funded clients was, in general, more readily available
- some surveys on the workforce in the independent sector were carried out nearly six years ago.

---

[1] We would like to thank colleagues at the PSSRU for their help in writing this appendix: Steve Almond, Julien Forder, Martin Knapp and Raphael Wittenberg. This appendix has been written in equal measure by Tihana Matosevic and Adelina Comas-Herrera. Jeremy Kendall wrote some of the introductory material in section one, as well as advising on content, data sources and definitions for the Appendix as a whole.

1   Size of the workforce

The total number of people employed in social care is officially reported to be 'around one million. This includes people working in a wide range of care settings, two-thirds of them in the independent sector (mainly working in residential homes)'.[2] (Department of Health, 1998)

There are essentially two routes to generating a 'global' estimate of paid employment in this field. One is to piece together specialist separate surveys from government and other sources, and aggregate them. This results in a figure of just over 900,000, as shown in Table 1.1. The second is to rely on the generic labour force survey (Quarterly Labour Force Survey, QFLS), which incidentally picks up paid employment in the 'social work industry' or part of the broader mapping of the entire workforce routinely undertaken by government.[3] (Almond and Kendall, 2000) This route generates a considerably higher figure of 1.18 million in 1998, including 467,900 in 'social work with accommodation', 715,600 in 'social work without accommodation', and, cutting across these 'industries', the largest single occupation was 'care assistants and attendants', numbering 513,600.

Why do these figures differ? Most obviously, there are differences in the year to which the estimates relate, geographical area, and, especially in the specialist surveys, problems of response rate bias. Detailed deconstruction of the QLFS suggests the social work 'industry' include some workers who have been misclassified, or who do not easily fit anywhere, such as some voluntary sector employees working in other, non-social care welfare fields. This would suggest the QLFS provides an *overestimate* in terms of the coverage aimed for in the report. However, the QLFS figures reported here only include 'main jobs', and the exclusion of second jobs means that the figure tends towards an *underestimate* in terms of total employment. It has not proved possible to quantify the net effect of these contradictory influences.

---

[2] The figure of one million excludes informal carers and unpaid volunteers, whose crucial contribution to social care is discussed elsewhere in the body of this report.

[3] See sections below for more details of this data source, where it is used to analyse pay differentials and a number of other workforce characteristics.

In fact, the true figure is probably likely to be more than 1 million, because the gaps left by the specialist surveys seem unlikely to involve less than 40,000 additional staff. Thus, the QLFS is implicitly picking up a range of social care activities not included in the specialist surveys aggregated in Table 1.1. For example:

- In terms of client group, community-based services for homeless people, people with human immunodeficiency syndrome (HIV)/acquired immunodeficiency syndrome (AIDS), alcohol problems, and other smaller client groups, may not be systematically included. The surveys in Table 1.1 include only adult services.

- The social care input of public and for-profit sector sheltered, very sheltered (and similar) housing-based services are also omitted.

- Other gaps relate to people employed, particularly in the independent sector, to deliver low intensity forms of care, such as community workers and paid volunteer organisers (Quilgars D, 2000; Lewis *et al.*, 1999).

- Some people whose posts are in the grey area of departmental demarcation, including many jointly funded by social services departments (SSDs) and health authorities (and perhaps voluntary sector, or other public sector department, cross-subsidy)

- More generally, employment in the independent sectors, *other than* residential and domiciliary care should be taken into account. Some of this may be funded by SSDs (as with day care provided under contract by voluntary organisations), but other independent sector non-residential, non-domiciliary, social care may be funded through private fees or charitable support.

- The QFLS figure also implicitly includes staff employed in homes with less than four residents which, in general, have been omitted from the specialist surveys such as the LGMB.

Below, we examine the nature of this workforce in more detail, considering the data from a range of sources including: Department of Health (DoH) statistics, the Local Government Management Board (LGMB) *Independent sector workforce survey 1996*, and the Housing Corporation data on Registered Social Landlords (RSLs). Some or all of these seem to have been fed into the White Paper *Modernising Social Services* figure.

Table 1.1 Estimates of the care workforce in England

Type of care staff	Head count	Year	Source	Comment
Home care staff – independent sector	127,000	1998	UKHCA estimates and DoH returns SSDS001; published in Laing and Buisson (2000). *Domiciliary care markets 2000*	The DoH statistics are based on a return (SSDS001) that collects information on all staff directly employed by SSDs. See Table 1.6
Home care staff – local authority	74,000	1999	DoH (2001). Local authority staffing statistics. DoH web site	The DoH statistics are based on a return (SSDS001) that collects information on all staff directly employed by SSDs
Residential and nursing homes – independent sector	487,000	1996	Local Government Management Board (LGMB) (1997). *Independent sector workforce survey 1996. Residential and nursing homes in Great Britain*	The independent sector workforce survey was conducted by the LGMB between August 1996 and January 1997, including 2,791 homes with four or more beds. See Table 1.12
Residential and other staff – local authority (including strategic and central staff)	133,000	1999	DoH (2001). Local authority staffing statistics. DoH web site	See Table 1.2
Day care staff – local authority	35,000	1999	DoH (2001). Local authority staffing statistics. DoH web site	See Table 1.2
Health care assistants	27,500	2000	*NHS hospital and community health services non-medical staff in England: 1999–2000*; DoH Bulletin 2001/3	DoH Bulletin 2001/3
Sheltered housing wardens – 'social care' activities, RSL sector	19,100	1999	Housing Corporation data on RSLs (1999); HAR10/1 RSR Part A	See Table 1.21. Includes voluntary sector, omits public and private (for-profit) sectors
Total care staff	**902,600**			

Sources: DoH SSD, SSDS001 return, 1999; LGMB *Independent sector workforce survey 1996*; DoH HCHS staffing statistical bulletin, 1999; *NHS hospital and community health services non-medical staff in England: 1999–2000*, DoH Bulletin 2001/3; housing corporation data on RSLs, 1999.

Local authority staff

Table 1.2 Total number of staff working for local authorities providing services for adults, England, 1999

Type of care	Total number of persons
Residential care	69,736
Domiciliary care	73,963
Day care	34,911
Other settings (including strategic and central staff)	62,920
Total	**241,530**

Source: SSDS001 return, DoH web site

The greater use of the independent sector in providing social services has been paralleled by a reduced significance of local authority services as the trends in Table 1.3 demonstrate.

Table 1.3 Staff of local authority SSDs annually at 30 September, England

Staff location	Whole-time equivalent (thousands)					
	1994	1995	1996	1997	1998	1999
Area office/field work staff	117	117	116	115	112	111
Domiciliary (home care) staff	59	57	55	54	51	47
Residential care staff	72	69	68	65	62	59
Day care staff	31	31	32	31	30	31
Central/strategic HQ staff	15	15	16	16	17	19
Other staff	3	2	2	2	2	2
Total	**238**	**234**	**234**	**229**	**224**	**222**

Source: SSDS001 return, DoH Bulletin 2000/6

In September 1999, local authority SSDs in England employed 221,700 whole-time equivalent staff. This represents a drop of about 1 per cent in numbers employed by local authorities since September 1998 and 7 per cent since September 1994.

Just over a quarter of these staff are employed in residential care. However, there has been an 18 per cent fall in these numbers over the last five years. The figures in Table

1.3 indicate a 5 per cent fall in the whole-time equivalent staff working in residential care between 1998 and 1999 alone. This probably indicates greater use of the independent sector for residential care services.

At the same time, associated with the development of the commissioning and managing role of social services, there has been an expansion of staff employed in central and strategic roles, and the number of staff working in social services headquarters (HQ) rose by 7 per cent between 1998 and 1999 and 23 per cent between 1994 and 1999.

Area office staff and field work staff account for almost half of the whole-time equivalent workforce. The number of staff employed in the home care/home help services has fallen by 20 per cent over the last five years, and by 6 per cent between 1998 and 1999. This reflects the tendency of local SSDs to make greater use of the independent sector to provide home care.

Table 1.4 shows that over the period between 1994 and 1999 about 58 per cent of social services staff were employed on a part-time basis.

Table 1.4 Trend in full-time/part-time working in social services (including services for children) between 1994 and 1999, England

Full-time/part-time working	1994	1995	1996	1997	1998	1999
Full-time	135,300	132,300	131,700	128,800	125,100	125,400
Part-time	180,400	182,300	181,000	179,900	174,200	170,200
Percentage						
Full-time	43%	42%	42%	42%	42%	42%
Part-time	57%	58%	58%	58%	58%	58%
All staff	**315,700**	**314,600**	**312,700**	**308,700**	**299,300**	**295,700**

Source: SSDS001 return, DoH Bulletin 2000/6

As Table 1.5 indicates, part-time working is characteristic of care staff, thus while only around a quarter of managerial staff, social workers, care managers and day centre officers work part-time, around a half of all social services officers or social work assistants and occupational therapists work part-time, as do around three-quarters of care staff and other support services staff.

Nearly two-thirds (64 per cent) of all the staff employed in adult services by local authorities SSDs work part-time. The sector with the highest percentage of people working part-time is home care (90 per cent).

Table 1.5 Number of persons employed in local authority SSDs (except services for children), by position, England, 1998–9

Position	Total number of persons	% who work part-time
Managerial or supervisory staff	45,499	25.1
Social workers	8,667	28.4
Social services officers/social work assistants	1,684	40.8
Care managers	1,971	24.6
Occupational therapists	831	51.9
Care staff	52,668	76.5
Home carers/helps/wardens/meals services	67,110	90.0
Day centre officers	10,439	28.2
Other support services staff	52,661	65.3
Total	**241,530**	**63.6**

Source: Local authority staffing statistics, 1999, DoH web site

1.1 Home care staff

There were approximately 200,000 people working in the delivery, administration or management of domiciliary care in England in 1998. Sixty-two per cent of all home care staff were employed in the independent sector (Table 1.6).

Table 1.6 Numbers of staff employed in delivering and managing home care, England, 1998

Category	Persons employed
Local authority home care workers	70,000
Independent sector home care workers	117,000
Local authority home care managers	5,000
Independent sector home care managers	5,000
Local authority administrative staff	2,000
Independent sector administrative staff	5,000
Total	**204,000**

Sources: UKHCA estimates and DoH returns SSDS001. Published in Laing and Buisson (2000). *Domiciliary care markets 2000*

Table 1.7 Home care staff employed by social services departments, England, 1999

Position	Total number of staff	Whole-time equivalent
Home/domiciliary care/help organisers	2,605	2,359
Assistant and trainee home care/help organisers	2,263	1,884
Home care staff/home helps	64,446	39,774
Wardens	1,916	1,433
Meals services staff where separately identifiable	748	375
Support services staff	1,985	1,402
Total	**73,963**	**47,227**

Source: Local authority staffing statistics, 1999, DoH web site

1.2 Staff working in residential and nursing care homes

Table 1.8 shows that, in 1999, 87 per cent of the total care staff working in residential and nursing homes were employed in the independent sector.

Table 1.8 Staff employed in residential and nursing homes (independent and local authority), England, 1999

Staff location	Number of people
Staff in residential and nursing homes – independent sector	487,000
Staff in residential homes – local authority	70,000
Total	**557,000**

Sources: DoH, SSD Staffing Bulletin, 1999; LGMB, 1997; DoH HCHS staffing Statistical Bulletin, 1999

Table 1.9 Social services staff employed in homes for elderly people and elderly people with a mental infirmity, England, 1999

Position	Total number of staff	Whole-time equivalent
Managers and officers in charge	1,155	1,136
Deputy officers in charge	1,644	1,527
Other supervisory staff	3,467	2,858
Care staff	25,380	17,022
Other support services staff	12,196	7,181
Total	**43,842**	**29,724**

Source: Local authority staffing statistics, 1999, DoH web site

Table 1.10 Social services staff employed in homes and hostels mainly for adults with mental health problems and learning disabilities

Position	Total number of staff	Whole-time equivalent
Managers and officers in charge	688	675
Deputy officers in charge	865	818
Other supervisory staff	2,405	1,971
Care staff	11,225	8,215
Other support services staff	2,108	1,272
Total	**17,291**	**12,951**

Source: Local authority staffing statistics, 1999, DoH web site

More than half (58 per cent) of the total social services staff working in residential homes for elderly people in 1999 were care staff. Only 3 per cent of social services staff employed in provision of residential care were managers and officers in charge (Table 1.9).

Similarly, care staff account for nearly two-thirds (65 per cent) of the total social services staff working in residential homes for adults with mental health and learning disabilities. The figures in Table 1.10 show that only 4 per cent were officers in charge and managers.

Table 1.11 Independent sector staff employed in residential homes in England, 1996 – workforce estimates

Number of homes	12,725
Registered beds	247,141
Nursing and care staff	
Full-time	93,200
Part-time	94,200
Total number	187,400
Total full-time equivalent	141,300
Other staff	
Full-time	14,900
Part-time	41,600
Total number	56,500
Total full-time equivalent (FTE)	34,700
Casual staff (full-time)	6,900
Agency staff (full-time)	1,400
Bank staff (FTE)	1,600
Grand total	
Total number of staff	252,100
Total number of FTE	185,800

Source: LGMB (1997) *Independent sector workforce survey 1996*

Table 1.12 indicates the relatively low proportion of staff employed in managerial and supervisory positions in care homes relative to the numbers of hands-on care staff.

Table 1.12 Distribution of all staff by position and type of home, England, 1996 – total numbers of staff

Type of home	Number of staff	Proportion (%) of staff
Residential and dual registered homes		
Managers/supervisors	42,500	13.1
Nursing staff	20,800	6.4
Care assistants	168,500	51.9
Other care staff	8,200	2.5
All nursing/care staff (total)	240,000	73.9
Other staff	75,000	23.1
Bank staff	–	–
Agency staff	1,900	0.6
Casual staff	7,800	2.4
Nursing homes		
Managers/supervisors	11,200	6.9
Nursing staff	30,400	18.7
Care assistants	75,800	46.7
Other care staff	1,900	1.2
All nursing/care staff (total)	119,300	73.5
Other staff	39,800	24.5
Bank staff	–	–
Agency staff	1,500	0.9
Casual staff	1,700	1.0
Total	**487,000**	**100.0**

Source: LGMB independent sector workforce survey, 1996

1.3 Health care assistants

Health care assistants are defined as ' those staff who are trained, or under training in the various competencies related to their job. This training might be through NVQ or other local HCA training' (DoH 2001, Bulletin 2001/3).

The figures in Table 1.13 show that, in 2000, there were 27,500 health care assistants working in the NHS and community health services. The majority of health care assistants (61 per cent) worked in the acute, elderly and general area of work. Table 1.14 shows that only 1,054 health care assistants were employed in community health services.

Table 1.13 Number of health care assistants working in the NHS and community health services (head count), England

	1995	1996	1997	1998	1999	2000
Health care assistants	16,240	20,220	21,500	24,630	25,470	27,500

Source: NHS hospital and community health services non-medical staff in England, DoH Bulletin 2001/3

Table 1.14 Number of health care assistants working in Community Health Services, England, 2000 (head count)

Health care assistants in community health services	1,054
Total no of health care assistants	27,500

Source: DoH. Non-medical workforce census, 2001

1.4 Support workers in other settings

Local authority staff employed in provision of day care services

Table 1.15 Staff employed in day centres mainly for elderly and people with a mental infirmity, England, 1999

Position	Total number of staff	Whole-time equivalent
Managers and officers in charge	404	382
Deputy officers in charge	256	229
Social work staff	48	35
Day centre officers	707	592
Care staff	2,531	1,662
Other support services staff	1,316	747
Total	**5,262**	**3,647**

Source: Local authority staffing statistics, 1999, DoH web site

Table 1.16 Staff employed in day centres mainly for adults with mental health problems and people with learning disabilities, England, 1999

Position	Total number of staff	Whole-time equivalent
Managers and officers in charge	860	835
Deputy officers in charge	910	857
Social work staff	370	319
Day centre officers	8,839	7,707
Care staff	4,143	2,989
Other support services staff	4,228	2,703
Total	**19,350**	**15,410**

Source: Local authority staffing statistics, 1999, DoH web site

Table 1.17 Staff employed in day centres for mixed client groups and people under 65 with physical disabilities, England, 1999

Position	Total number of staff	Whole-time equivalent
Managers and officers in charge	325	318
Deputy officers in charge	332	203
Social work staff	103	683
Day centre officers	1,627	1,332
Care staff	1,506	1,643
Other support services staff	2,189	3,293
Total	**6,082**	**7,472**

Source: Local authority staffing statistics, 1999, DoH web site

As Table 1.15 demonstrates, the number of care staff in day centres for elderly people and people with a mental infirmity accounts for almost half (48 per cent) of the total number of staff working with this client group. It is interesting to note that only 1 per cent were employed as social workers.

Table 1.16 shows that 46 per cent of staff providing day care for adults with mental health problems and people with learning disabilities were day centre officers and around 2 per cent of staff were working as social workers.

Similarly, figures in Table 1.17 indicate that more than one-third (36 per cent) of all staff in day centres for mixed client groups and people under 65 with physical disabilities were support staff, whereas only 2 per cent were social workers.

Other local authority services

Table 1.18 Staff in operational divisions/not establishment based, England, 1999

Position	Total number of staff	Whole-time equivalent
Team leaders/managers	1,151	1,099
Assistant team managers/senior social workers	824	742
Care managers	2,168	1,950
Field social workers	4,071	3,578
Social services officers/social work assistants	2,469	2,107
Community workers	737	585
Occupational therapists (OT)	1,183	916
OT assistants, equipment aids and other officers	881	739
Technical officers	224	193
Total	**13,708**	**11,909**

Source: Local authority staffing statistics, 1999, DoH web site

Table 1.18 shows that 30 per cent of staff in operational divisions were employed as field social workers followed by social services officers and social work assistants (18 per cent).

Table 1.19 Field social workers providing health-related social work, England, 1999

Position	Total number of staff	Whole-time equivalent
Team leaders/managers	444	411
Care managers	529	471
Social workers	2,476	2,119
Social services officers/social work assistants	556	482
Total	**4,005**	**3,483**

Source: Local authority staffing statistics, 1999, DoH web site

Table 1.20 Specialist teams in alcohol, HIV/AIDS and drug centres, England, 1999

Position	Total number of staff	Whole-time equivalent
Team leaders/managers	94	83
Assistant managers/senior social workers	63	59
Social workers	262	230
Care managers in alcohol, HIV/AIDS and drug centres	85	75
Support workers	66	58
Total	**570**	**505**

Source: Local authority staffing statistics, 1999, DoH web site

Table 1.21 Other specialist teams (e.g. mental health, people with learning disabilities and/or physical disabilities)

Position	Total number of staff	Whole-time equivalent
Team leaders/managers	811	772
Assistant managers/senior social workers	782	737
Social workers	3,914	3,496
Care managers in specialist teams for mental health	1,056	941
Support workers	1,958	1,539
Total	**8,521**	**7,485**

Source: Local authority staffing statistics, 1999, DoH web site

The figures in Tables 1.19–1.21 indicate that around 50 per cent of the staff working with these client groups were social workers.

1.5 Sheltered housing wardens and other housing support staff

We were unable to trace data on the numbers of sheltered housing wardens employed by local authorities in delivering social care or otherwise. Neither were data available for the private (for-profit) sector. However, information on the numbers of care staff employed by RSLs (voluntary sector) was supplied to us by the Housing Corporation. This is shown in Table 1.22.

Table 1.22 Care staff employed by RLSs (registered social landlords) between 1997 and 1999

Full-time equivalent	1997	1998	1999
Care staff	17,100	16,500	19,100

Source: Housing Corporation data on RSLs 1999; HAR10/1 RSR Part A

Note: 'Care staff' category includes staff providing personal care, advice, and wardens in supported housing.

2   Profile of the workforce

2.1 Age and gender breakdown

The QLFS is the most comprehensive nationally representative survey of employment in the UK. Its sample consists of more than 60,000 households interviewed every quarter. The data from the QLFS presented here comes from a study of the quality of UK third-sector employment (Almond and Kendall, 2000) where data were pooled from four quarters during 1998 (Winter 1997 to Autumn 1998). A care occupations sub-sample has been selected, encompassing care assistants, social workers, nurses, occupational therapists, assistant nurses and auxiliaries, cleaners and other domestics.

As Table 2.1 shows, around 30 per cent of all people in the QLFS care occupations sub-sample were aged 50 years or over, with rising proportions of people in each subsequent age group.

Table 2.1 QLFS (care occupations sub-sample): percentage of staff in each age group

Age group	Percentage (%)
Under 30 years	19.3
30–39 years	23.6
40–49 years	26.3
50 years or more	30.8

Source: Based on Almond and Kendal (2000)

A very similar age distribution was found in the UKHCA survey (Mathew, 2000) of domiciliary care workers in the independent sector:

Table 2.2 Age of domiciliary care workers

Age group	% of workers (n = 1278)
Under 30 years	19
30–39 years	24
40–49 years	25
50 years and over	32

Source: Mathew (2000)

Gender

Table 2.3 shows that nearly 89 per cent of staff in the QLFS care occupations sub-sample were female. There is not a marked variation in gender for the different age groups. At most, it appears that there is a slightly higher proportion of males in the age group 30 to 39, compared to other age groups, and a slightly lower proportion of males in the group over 50 years old.

Table 2.3 Gender by age, in percentages

Age group	Male	Female	% of total by age group
Under 30 years	11.2	88.8	19.3
30–39 years	14.9	85.1	23.6
40–49 years	11.7	88.3	26.3
50 years or more	8.1	91.9	30.8
% of total by gender	11.2	88.8	100

Source: Based on Almond and Kendal (2000)

Local authority sector

Table 2.4 shows that in 1998–9 in England, 86 per cent of the local authority social services workforce was female. Of those, only 31 per cent were working full-time, whereas most men (74 per cent) were working full-time.

Almost all (97 per cent) home carers, home helps, wardens and people involved in meals services are female and work part-time. In contrast, whereas nearly 92 per cent of occupational therapists are female, only 52 per cent of them work part-time. This seems to indicate that although gender is a clear predictor of part-time working, women are most likely to work part-time in jobs requiring few qualifications.

Table 2.4 Number of persons employed in local authority SSDs (except services for children), by position, England, 1998–9

Position	Total number of staff	% who are females	% who are part-time	% of females who work part-time	% of part-time people who are females
Managerial or supervisory staff	45,499	77.2	25.1	29.7	91.5
Social workers	8,667	73.7	28.4	34.0	88.1
Social services officers/social work assistants	1,684	79.8	40.8	44.1	86.2
Care managers	1,971	76.0	24.6	28.9	89.3
Occupational therapists	831	91.9	51.9	54.8	97.2
Care staff	52,668	88.5	76.5	79.5	92.0
Home carers/helps, wardens, meals services	67,110	97.3	90.0	90.7	97.9
Day centre officers	10,439	68.6	28.2	34.5	84.0
Other support services staff	52,661	82.1	65.3	70.1	88.1
Total	**241,530**	**85.9**	**63.6**	**69.0**	**93.2**

Source: Local authority staffing statistics, 1999, DoH web site

Independent sector

The 1996 independent sector workforce survey of residential and nursing homes in Great Britain (LGMB, 1997) found that the proportion of females working in residential and nursing homes was around 90 per cent (Table 2.11).

Working part-time: the reasons

Reasons for working part-time may reflect a complex interaction of choice and circumstances. The QLFS asked people who worked part-time why they did so. Among those in the care occupations sub-sample of the QLFS who worked part-time, the vast majority (81 per cent) said that they did not want a full-time job. Fourteen per cent said they could not find a full-time job.

Table 2.5 Reason for working part-time

Reason	Percentages
Student or at school	3.8
Ill or disabled	1.1
Could not find a full-time job	14.2
Did not want a full-time job	80.9

Source: Based on Almond and Kendall (2000)

2.2 Data on ethnic composition

The social services workforce surveys are carried out by the Employment Surveys and Research Unit (ESRU) of the Employers Organisation (EO) for local government and commissioned by the Social and Health Care Workforce Group (formerly by the LGMB/ADSS). Data were collected in 1997, 1998 and 1999 on the gender, ethnicity, qualifications and recruitment and retention of employees of local authority social services, by looking at different parts of the workforce every year.[4]

---

[4] The 1997 survey concentrated on some area social services groups and staff in mental health and children's residential care settings. The 1998 survey concentrated on other area social services groups, day care and residential care staff and approved social workers. Finally, the 1999 survey focussed on: social services officers, community workers, occupational therapists (OT), OT assistants, home care organisers (Wales only), home carers (Wales only), staff in day centres (for elderly people, people under 65 with physical disabilities, adults with mental health problems, adults with learning disabilities and mixed client groups), family centres and day nurseries. These data were provided by between 62 and 69 authorities (depending on job category).

Table 2.6 Comparison of the ethnicity of social services workforce surveys groups with the whole QLFS population of working age, England

Percentages	1997		1998		1999	
	Social services workforce survey	QLFS (population aged 16–64)	Social services workforce survey	QLFS (population aged 16–64)	Social services workforce survey	QLFS (population aged 16–64)
Bangladeshi	0.1	0.3	0.0	0.4	0.2	0.5
Black African	3.0	0.7	1.4	0.7	1.6	0.7
Black Caribbean	3.7	1.1	3.0	1.0	3.2	1.1
Black Other	1.9	0.2	0.8	0.2	0.8	0.4
Chinese	0.1	0.4	0.1	0.4	0.1	0.3
Indian	1.5	2.0	0.7	2.1	1.7	2.0
Pakistani	0.4	1.1	1.4	1.1	0.7	1.2
Irish	1.2	92.6	1.3	92.5	0.7	92.7
White	85.6		89.5		88.3	
Other	2.5	1.5	1.7	1.5	2.5	1.2
Base (numbers)	**41,191**	**31,078,378**	**138,910**	**31,179,642**	**41,492**	**29,225,104**

Source: Social Services Workforce Survey Report, 1997,1998, 1999

For all three workforce surveys, the proportion of white people (including Irish) in the social services groups covered by the survey is lower than the population of working age as a whole. Whereas the proportions of black African, black Caribbean and black Other are higher among the social services staff sample than among the working age population, Asian people are under-represented. The differences between the three years of the social services workforce survey are likely to be due to the different employment groups targeted in each of the years. It is unlikely to be due to changes over time, because there are no observable trends in the QLFS.

As Table 2.7 shows, the UKHCA survey (2000) found a lower proportion of domiciliary care workers from ethnic minority backgrounds (6.5 per cent), which is closer to the proportion observed in the LFS sample. However, the UKHCA survey figure is likely to be an under-estimate because the response rate for London and other metropolitan areas was low, and these are precisely the areas where the proportion of home care workers from ethnic minority groups is much higher.

Table 2.7 Ethnic origin of domiciliary care staff

Ethnic origin	Percent of workers (n = 1281)
Asian	0.9
Black	3.7
Mixed	0.9
Other	0.9
White	93.5

Source: Mathew (2000)

2.3 Variations

Geographical variations and ethnicity

The social services workforce surveys found variation in the ethnic background of staff between different types of authority. London boroughs employ the highest proportion of people from ethnic minorities. Metropolitan districts employ the second highest proportion, while a low proportion of people from ethnic minorities are employed in the counties and unitary authorities, reflecting the characteristics of the overall population in the different types of local authorities. Table 2.8 shows as an example[5] the ethnicity of staff in homes for elderly people in England, 1998, by type of local authority.

---

[5] We are unable to present a table for the overall sector from the data available in the workforce survey report.

Table 2.8 Ethnicity of staff in homes for elderly people in England, 1998, by type of local authority

Ethnicity	Homes for elderly people							
	Officers in charge/deputies/other supervisory staff (percentages)				Care staff (percentages)			
	LB	MD	C	UA	LB	MD	C	UA
Bangladeshi	0.0	0.3	0.0	0.0	0.0	0.0	0.0	0.1
Black African	2.7	2.7	0.1	0.9	9.3	2.2	0.3	0.2
Black Caribbean	19.8	6.1	0.6	1.2	17.1	5.0	0.4	2.3
Black Other	0.9	0.1	0.1	0.9	3.1	0.5	0.2	0.7
Chinese	0.0	0.0	0.2	0.3	0.0	0.0	0.1	0.1
Indian	0.0	1.0	0.3	0.0	2.5	1.4	0.7	0.7
Irish	2.7	0.3	0.1	4.4	6.2	0.2	0.0	2.6
Pakistani	0.0	0.4	0.0	0.3	0.6	0.7	0.0	0.3
White	65.8	87.5	96.1	91.0	56.2	87.5	96.1	92.1
Other	8.1	1.8	2.3	0.9	5.0	2.4	2.1	0.9
Total employment	**713**	**1,596**	**3,133**	**1,540**	**2,937**	**6,679**	**13,678**	**5,454**

Source: Social and Health Care Workforce Group (1999). *Social services workforce analysis 1998. Main report.* Based on responses from 6–9 London boroughs (LB), 20–24 metropolitan districts (MD), 14–21 counties (C) and 16–22 unitary authorities (UA)

Variations of gender according to occupation

As Tables 2.9–2.11 indicate, the social care workforce is typically female, and this is especially the case with front line care staff.

Table 2.9 QLFS, percentages of men and women, by occupation

Occupation	Men	Women
Social workers, probation officers	33.4	66.6
Nurses	11.3	88.7
Occupational and speech therapists	9.3	90.7
Assistant nurses and auxiliaries	17.4	82.6
Care assistants and attendants	6.6	93.4
Cleaners, domestics	3.7	96.7
Total	**11.2**	**88.8**

Source: Based on Almond and Kendal (2000)

Local authority sector

Table 2.10 Number of persons employed in local authority SSDs (except services for children), by position, England, 1998–9

Position	Total number of staff	% who are females
Managerial or supervisory staff	45,499	77.2
Social workers	8,667	73.7
Social services officers/ social work assistants	1,684	79.8
Care managers	1,971	76.0
Occupational therapists	831	91.9
Care staff	52,668	88.5
Home carers/helps/wardens/ Meals services	67,110	97.3
Day centre officers	10,439	68.6
Other support services staff	52,661	82.1
Total	**241,530**	**85.9**

Source: Calculated from data available from the DoH web site

3   Total expenditure on care and support work

Overall expenditure, public and private

The PSSRU long-term care financing model (Wittenberg *et al.*, 1998) produces projections of the future demand and expenditure on long-term care services for older people in England.

In 1996, the estimated total expenditure on long-term care services for older people was nearly £10 billion. As Table 3.1 shows, using the model's base case assumptions, expenditure in real terms is expected to have risen to £10.5 billion by 2000 and to £24 billion by 2031 to keep apace with demographic trends. If the same system of long-term care financing remained in place, the share of expenditure borne by the recipients of services would be expected to rise from 35 per cent in 1996 to 37 per cent in 2031.

Table 3.1 Expenditure in long-term care for older people by source: 1996 figures and projections from the PSSRU long-term care financing model (billions of pounds)

Expenditure source	1996	2000	2010	2020	2031
NHS	2.2	2.3	2.9	4.0	6.0
PSS net	4.3	4.4	5.1	6.5	9.3
Total public finance	6.4	6.8	8.1	10.5	15.3
User fees	1.5	1.5	1.8	2.3	3.4
Private sector	1.9	2.2	3.0	3.8	5.6
Total private finance	3.4	3.7	4.8	6.1	9.0
Overall expenditure	9.8	10.5	12.8	16.6	24.3

Source: Wittenberg *et al.* (2001), using the PSSRU long-term care financing model

Projected increases in the demand for long-term care services older people

Table 3.2 Estimated increase in the volume of services for older people required in England, according to the base case of the PSSRU long-term care financing model (in 1000s)

Service	2000	2010	2031	% increase 2000 to 2010	% increase 2000 to 2031
Home help (hours/visits)	1,938	2,029	2,901	4.69	49.7
Community nurse (hours/visits)	657	712	1,063	8.51	61.9
Day centre (hours/visits)	213	222	321	4.66	50.9
Private domestic help (hours/visits)	891	994	1,472	11.59	65.2
Meals-on-wheels (hours/visits)	732	798	1,143	9.06	56.2
Luncheon club (hours/visits)	360	385	556	7.02	54.6
Chiropody (hours/visits)	353	381	566	7.95	60.4
Residential homes (residents)	252	274	398	8.50	57.9
Nursing homes (residents)	138	151	225	9.04	63.0

Source: Calculated using the PSSRU long-term care financing model

Table 3.3 shows the impact on the future volume of services for the elderly required (using the PSSRU long-term care financing model projections for England) if people who have informal carers are given the same care packages as those who do not have informal carers (in other words, if the care packages were carer-blind; see Pickard *et al.* (2000) for more details).

Table 3.3 Estimated increase in the future volume of services for the elderly required if care packages were carer-blind (1000s)

Service	2000	2031 base case	2031 carer-blind	% increase 2000 to 2031 base case	% increase 2000 to 2031 carer- blind
Home help (hours/visits)	1,938	2,901	3,500	49.7	80.6
Community nurse (hours/visits)	657	1063	1,063	61.9	61.9
Day centre (hours/visits)	213	321	368	50.9	73.1
Private domestic help (hours/visits)	891	1472	1,637	65.2	83.8
Meals-on-wheels (hours/visits)	732	1143	1,528	56.2	108.7
Luncheon club (hours/visits)	360	556	659	54.6	83.2
Chiropody (hours/visits)	353	566	566	60.4	60.4

Source: Pickard *et al.* (2000) using the PSSRU long-term care financing model

Other estimates of overall expenditure

The figures presented above only refer to the demand and expenditure for older people in England. Laing and Buisson (2000) in their latest *Care of Elderly People Market Survey 2000* have estimated the market value[6] of the care for elderly, chronically ill and physically disabled people in 2000 in the UK was £13.2 billion. Of this, £8.6 billion was represented by residential care and £4.6 billion by non-residential care (Table 3.4).

---

[6] Laing and Buisson calculate market value as the number of beds multiplied by fee levels for residential settings. For non-residential services they calculate it using DoH expenditure data as well as Laing and Buisson data on personal expenditure on home care.

Table 3.4 Nursing and residential care of elderly, chronically ill and physically disabled people: annual market value annualised at April 2000, UK

Type of nursing and reisdential care	£ million
Private nursing	3,248
Private residential	2,349
Total private (for-profit) supply	5,597
Voluntary nursing	367
Voluntary residential	764
Total voluntary (not-for-profit) supply	1,131
NHS long stay geriatric	594
NHS elderly mentally ill	358
NHS younger physically disabled	44
Local authority elderly and younger physically disabled	890
Total public supply	1,886
Total care in residential settings	8,614
Non-residential care	4,597
Grand total	13,208

Source: Laing and Buisson (2000). *Care of elderly people market survey 2000*, p. 21

Local authority expenditure

The gross expenditure by local authority SSDs in England in 1998–9 was £10.8 billion. This figure includes expenditure on services for children, as well as for elderly people and chronically ill and physically disabled adults. There has been a steady increase in expenditure in the last decade, from £5.6 billion in 1988–9, to £10.8 in ten years.

Table 3.5 Gross local authority expenditure in social services in England

Year	Gross expenditure (in 1998–9 prices, £ million)
1988–9	5,600
1989–90	5,800
1990–1	6,100
1991–2	6,200
1992–3	6,400
1993–4	7,200
1994–5	8,500
1995–6	9,200
1996–7	9,800
1997–8	10,300
1998–9	10,800

Source: DoH (2000). *Personal social services current expenditure in England: 1998–9*. Statistical Bulletin 2000/10

3.1 Breakdown of expenditure between types of services (domiciliary care, including community nursing/joint schemes; care homes; day services; sheltered housing; other supported housing, etc.)

Local authority expenditure by client group and type of service

Of the £10.8 billion gross expenditure by local authorities in England in 1998–9, 48 per cent was spent on older people, 23 per cent on children, 7 per cent on physically disabled people, 14 per cent on people with learning difficulties and 5 per cent on people with mental health problems. 0.6 per cent was spent on people with HIV/AIDS or who are alcohol/drugs misusers, and 1.4 per cent was spent on service strategy and regulation.

Table 3.6 Personal social services current expenditure in England by client group, 1998–9 (£ million)

Type of PSS expenditure	Gross expenditure	% of total gross expenditure
Central/strategic	150	1.4
Children	2,470	22.8
Elderly people	5,220	48.1
People with a physical disability	750	6.9
People with learning disabilities	1,490	13.7
HIV and AIDS, drugs and alcohol misuse	60	0.6
People with mental health needs	560	5.2
Other	140	1.3
Total	**10,850**	**100**

Source: DoH web site

By type of provision, 48 per cent of gross local authority expenditure in 1998–9 was spent on residential care, 36 per cent on day care, 11 per cent on care management and social work, and 5 per cent on senior management and purchasing.

Table 3.7 Local authority personal social services expenditure by client group and type of service, 1998–99, England, £ million

Type of PSS expenditure	Elderly	Children	Learning disability	Physical disability	Mental health	Other	Total
HQ costs	–	–	–	–	–	149	149
Area officers/senior managers	103	161	26	29	28	–	348
Care management/care assessment	329	505	76	101	126	–	1,136
Residential care	3,180	724	838	218	224	–	5,184
Non–residential care	1,605	1,074	555	402	186	–	3,822
Other	–	–	–	–	–	208	208
Total	**5,220**	**2,470**	**1,490**	**750**	**560**	**360**	**10,850**

Source: DoH web site

Day and domiciliary provision

Table 3.8 presents estimates of the gross expenditure on non-residential community care services for elderly and physically disabled people. This includes estimates of privately purchased home care.

Table 3.8 Gross expenditure on non-residential community care services for elderly and physically disabled people, UK estimates by source of funding 1998/1999

NHS expenditure on non-residential care (community health)	£ million
Community nursing (non-psychiatric)	1,347
Chiropody	111
Day care (non-psychiatric)	141
Total NHS expenditure on non-residential care	1,599
Local authority expenditure on non-residential care (gross of user charges)	
Home care/home help	1,422
Day centres	318
Meals	94
Equipment and adaptations	77
Occupational therapy services	72
Direct payments	11
Other non-residential services	429
Total gross local authority expenditure on non-residential community care	2,423
Personal expenditure on private non-residential care (excluding user charges for local authority services)	
Home care purchased from home care businesses and non-profit providers	125
Home care purchased in the 'grey' economy	300
Aids and adaptations	150
Total personal expenditure	575
Total public and personal expenditure on non-residential care	4,597

Source: Laing and Buisson (2000). *Care of Elderly People Market Survey 2000*, p. 25. Personal expenditure on home care businesses extrapolated to 1999 from the results of a national sample survey of home care providers carried out by Laing and Buisson in 1997

Local authority

Table 3.9 shows expenditure on local authority day and domiciliary services, by client group.

Table 3.9 Day and domiciliary provision in England: main items of local authority expenditure 1997–8 and 1998–9, £ million

Category	1997–8		1998–9	
	Gross	Net	Gross	Net
Children				
– Foster placements	350	350	370	370
– Family centres/family support and under-8 provision	250	240	250	240
– Other (incl. administration)	350	350	450	450
Total	950	940	1,070	1,060
Elderly people				
– Day centres	170	150	180	160
– Home care/help	1,020	900	1,050	910
– Other (incl. administration)	360	300	370	320
Total	1,540	1,350	1,600	1,390
People with physical disabilities	380	360	400	380
People with learning disabilities	490	460	560	520
People with HIV and AIDS, alcohol or drugs misuse	10	10	.	.
People with mental health needs	170	170	190	180
Other	10	10	.	.
Total expenditure	**3,550**	**3,300**	**3,820**	**3,530**

Source: DoH web site

'.' denotes data not available.

Residential care

Table 3.10 shows the estimated value in the UK of the market in residential care for elderly, chronically ill and physically disabled people. In the last ten years, the balance of the provision of residential care between the public and the independent sector has shifted dramatically, with the independent sector gaining significance as a provider and as a major employer. In 1988, the public sector provision represented more than half of the total market value, whereas it represented less than a quarter by 1998–9. Most of this loss in the public sector market share has been compensated by growth in the for-profit sector, which grew from a 38 per cent market share in 1988 to 65 per cent in 1998–9.

Table 3.10 Nursing, residential and long-stay hospital care of elderly, chronically ill and physically disabled people, market value by sector to which the providers belong, UK 1988–2000 (annualised at April 2000), £ million

Year	Private sector	Private sector provision as % of total	Voluntary sector	Voluntary sector provision as % of total	Public sector (local authority homes and NHS units)	Public sector provision as % of total	Total
1988	1,734	38.4	433	9.6	2,344	52.0	4,5
1989	2,243	43.3	457	8.8	2,477	47.8	5,1
1990	2,704	46.3	471	8.1	2,661	45.6	5,8
1991	3,436	51.7	535	8.1	2,673	40.2	6,6
1992	3,939	54.7	659	9.1	2,609	36.2	7,2
1993	4,470	56.3	843	10.6	2,620	33.0	7,9
1994	4,683	58.1	926	11.5	2,453	30.4	8,0
1995	4,935	59.6	984	11.9	2,364	28.5	8,2
1996	5,044	60.8	996	12.0	2,262	27.2	8,3
1997	5,158	62.0	1,027	12.3	2,139	25.7	8,3
1998	5,322	63.1	1,057	12.5	2,054	24.4	8,4
1999	5,411	64.2	1,053	12.5	1,966	23.3	8,4
2000 (proj.)	5,597	65.0	1,131	13.1	1,886	21.9	8,6

Source: Laing and Buisson (2000). *Care of Elderly People Market Survey 2000*, p. 23

A similar picture emerges for the residential care services for people with mental illness and learning disabilities, as shown in Tables 3.11–3.13.

Table 3.11 Public/private mix of psychiatric rehabilitation and long-term nursing/residential care for mentally ill people, England, 1998

Public/private mental health	£ million
NHS mental health hospitals	276
Private non-acute nursing homes	92
Voluntary non-acute nursing homes	27
Psychiatric rehabilitation in private and voluntary psychiatric hospitals	70
Total nursing care	465
Local authority staffed premises	34
Private residential homes	140
Voluntary residential homes	71
Total residential care	245
Total nursing and residential expenditure	710

Source: Laing and Buisson (2000). *Healthcare market review 1999–2000*

Table 3.12 Public/private mix of long-term care nursing and residential care for people with learning disabilities, England, 1998

Public/private learning disabilities	£ million
NHS mental handicap hospitals	327
Private nursing homes	51
Voluntary nursing homes	37
Total nursing care	415
Local authority staffed homes	183
Private residential homes	431
Voluntary residential homes	341
Total residential care	955
Total nursing and residential care expenditure	1,370

Source: Laing and Buisson (2000). *Healthcare market review 1999–2000*

Table 3.13 Residential provision in England: main categories of expenditure by local authorities, 1997–8 and 1998–9, £ million

Category	Gross expenditure		Net expenditure	
	1997–8	1998–9	1997–8	1998–9
Children				
– Community homes	450	460	450	460
– Special education	60	70	60	70
– Children in secure accommodation	40	50	20	30
– Other (incl. admin)	140	150	140	140
Total	690	720	670	700
Elderly people				
– Own LA provision[1]	770	740	560	530
– Commissioned placements	970	1,170	550	640
– Nursing placements				
– Other (incl. admin)	950	1,020	640	670
Total	240	240	240	230
	2,940	3,180	1,980	2,080
People with physical disabilities	200	220	150	160
People with learning disabilities	740	840	570	620
People with HIV and AIDS, alcohol or drugs misuse[2]	20	.	10	.
People with mental health needs	210	220	150	160
Other	–	.	–	.
Total expenditure	**4,800**	**5,180**	**3,540**	**3,730**

Source: DoH web site

[1] Own local authority provision for 1997–8 includes placements in other local authorities.

[2] Not available for 1998–9.

'–' denotes a value less than £5 million.

'.' denotes data not available.

As Table 3.13 indicates, much of local authorities' expenditure on residential care is accounted for not by direct provision of care, but by commissioning placements in independent sector homes.

3.2 Proportion of public expenditure costs which are recovered through charges

The overall percentage of local authority social services expenditure recovered through charges in 1998–9 in England was 16.5 per cent. There are wide variations in the percentages recovered by the different authorities. The local authority with the lowest recovery rate recovered 0.1 per cent of its gross expenditure, and the highest recovered 32 per cent (DoH web site). There are also striking differences between client groups, with the highest proportion of expenditure recovered from charges to elderly people. This reflects the fact that elderly people are more likely to have accumulated savings and capital throughout their lives that are then drawn on through means-testing to fund part or all of their care.

Table 3.14 Percentage of gross expenditure recovered in fees and charges in England, 1998–9 by client group

Type of expenditure (client group)	% recovery in fees and charges
Central/strategic	11.4
Children	2.0
Elderly people	25.2
People with a physical disability	10.1
People with learning disabilities	16.9
HIV and AIDS, drugs and alcohol misuse	7.5
People with mental health needs	12.1
Other	2.2
Total	**16.5**

Source: Aggregated from data from the DoH web site

Table 3.15 Childrens services: percentage of gross expenditure recovered in charges, by type of service, England, 1998–9

Type of expenditure (children)	% recovery in fees and charges
Assessment and commissioning	0.4
Residential care	3.9
Non-residential services	1.8
Total childrens services	2.0

Source: Aggregated from data from the DoH web site

Table 3.16 Elderly and elderly mentally ill services: percentage of gross expenditure recovered in charges, by type of service, England, 1998–9

Type of expenditure (eldery and elderly mental ill)	% of recovery in fees and charges
Assessment and commissioning	1.0
Residential care placements: own local authority provision	28.2
Residential care placements: commissioned placements	45.1
Nursing placements	34.5
Other residential services for elderly	22.8
Total residential costs	**34.6**
Home care/home help	13.3
Day centres	11.0
Other non-residential costs	23.0
Total non-residential services	**13.2**
Total elderly and elderly mentally ill	**25.2**

Source: Aggregated from data from the DoH web site

Table 3.17 Physically disabled adults (under 65) services: percentage of gross expenditure recovered in charges, by type of service, England, 1998–9

Type of expenditure (physically disabled adults)	% recovery in fees and charges
Assessment and commissioning	0.6
Residential placement: own local authority provision	18.3
Residential placement: commissioned placements	29.0
Nursing placements	26.3
Other residential costs	4.1
Total residential costs	**24.8**
Home care/home help	7.7
Day centres	6.6
Other non-residential costs	3.4
Total non-residential costs	**5.3**
Total services for physically disabled adults	**10.1**

Source: Aggregated from data from the DoH web site

Table 3.18 Learning disabled adults (under 65) services: percentage of gross expenditure recovered in charges, by type of service, England, 1998–9

Type of expenditure (learning disabled adults)	% recovery in fees and charges
Assessment and commissioning	0.5
Residential placement: own local authority provision	23.4
Residential placement: commissioned placements	29.8
Nursing placements	22.9
Other residential costs	21.3
Total residential costs	**25.6**
Home care/home help	10.8
Day centres	6.0
Other non-residential costs	11.2
Total non-residential costs	**6.7**
Total services for learning disabled adults	**16.9**

Source: Aggregated from data from the DoH web site

Table 3.19 Adult mental health services: percentage of gross expenditure recovered in charges, by type of service, England, 1998–9

Type of expenditure (mental health)	% of recovery in fees and charges
Assessment and commissioning	1.3
Residential placement: own local authority provision	34.2
Residential placement: commissioned placements	29.6
Nursing placements	24.0
Other residential costs	17.3
Total residential costs	**27.3**
Home care/home help	6.0
Day centres	3.0
Other non-residential costs	2.1
Total non-residential costs	**2.9**
Total services for mental health	**12.1**

Source: Aggregated from data from the DoH web site

Trends over time on recovery of personal social services (PSS) expenditure

The percentage of gross expenditure recovered by local authorities has increased substantially from around 11 per cent in 1988–9 to nearly 16 per cent in 1998–9.

Table 3.20 Historical trends in gross and net PSS expenditure and percentage recovered by local authorities from 1988–9 to 1998–9 (£ million)

Year	Gross (in 1998–9 prices)	Net (in 1998–9 prices)	% of gross expenditure recovered
1988–9	5,600	5,000	10.7
1989–90	5,800	5,200	10.3
1990–1	6,100	5,400	11.5
1991–2	6,200	5,600	9.7
1992–3	6,400	5,800	9.4
1993–4	7,200	6,500	9.7
1994–5	8,500	7,500	11.8
1995–6	9,200	8,000	8.7
1996–7	9800	8,400	14.3
1997–8	10,300	8,700	15.5
1998–9	10,800	9,100	15.7

Source: DoH (2000). *PSS current expenditure in England: 1998–9.* Statistical Bulletin 2000/10

The Audit Commission survey of home care charging policy and practice across 140 councils in England and Wales (Audit Commission, 2000) found that the majority of councils charged for home care services and that most of them based the charges on the intensity of services received by the user and their means.

Table 3.21 Patterns of charging for home care (main approaches by local authorities)

Charging approach	% of LAs
Do not charge	6
Charge most users the same	10
Base charges on level of service	19
Base charges on a user's means	10
Base charges on both service and means	55

Source: Audit Commission (2000), p. 28

3.3 Variations between local authorities in price per hour paid for care services

Residential care

As the tables below show, there is a marked difference between the average weekly prices of residential care services between London and the rest of the country.

Table 3.22 Average gross weekly prices (£): independent sector (for-profit and voluntary) by care type

Authority type	Nursing	Residential	All
London	413	295	353
Metropolitan	312	223	263
Shire	324	230	270
All	334	237	280

Source: Netten *et al.* (1999), p. 97

Table 3.23 Average weekly fees, for-profit homes (March 2000)

Region	Nursing care		Residential care	
	Single	Shared	Single	Shared
North	334	333	248	240
Yorkshire and Humberside	350	333	249	239
North West	369	355	255	251
East Midlands	353	333	254	246
West Midlands	361	338	266	255
Northern Home Counties	460	409	343	294
East Anglia	378	366	273	257
Greater London	492	441	360	327
Southern Home Counties	435	371	304	271
South West	372	343	268	253
Wales	344	338	247	241
Scotland	375	342	275	256
Northern Ireland	344	339	235	228
United Kingdom	377	351	271	256

Source: Laing and Buisson (2000). *Care of elderly people market survey 2000*

Home care

Data on the variations in cost per hour of domiciliary services are available from a study of independent sector domiciliary care providers conducted as part of the Mixed Economy of Care Research programme (MEOC, jointly undertaken at the PSSRU, LSE, and Nuffield Institute for Health, University of Leeds).

The figures in the tables below show that prices for both practical and personal care were higher in London and the South. However, between 1995 and 1999 there was a higher rate of increase in the mean prices in the Northern authorities than in London and the South for both practical and personal care services (increases of 32 per cent and 17 per cent, respectively).

Table 3.24 Ranges of prices for practical care in 1995 and 1999 for local authority funded clients (weekdays)

Region	1995			1999		
	Practical care (£)			Practical care (£)		
	Mean	Minimum	Maximum	Mean	Minimum	Maximum
London and South	£6.89	£3.70	£13.60	£8.08	£5.00	£13.60
North	£5.22	£3.95	£7.50	£7.11	£4.50	£15.00

Source: Ware *et al.* (2001)

Table 3.25 Ranges of prices for personal care in 1995 and 1999 for local authority funded clients (weekdays)

Region	1995			1999		
	Personal care (£)			Personal care (£)		
	Mean	Minimum	Maximum	Mean	Minimum	Maximum
London and South	£7.21	£4.05	£13.60	£8.41	£5.00	£13.60
North	£5.35	£3.95	£7.50	£7.21	£4.98	£15.00

Source: Ware *et al.* (2001)

3.4 Self-paying, i.e. individuals making their own financial arrangements directly with service providers (and extent to which this is changing, and scope for more self-payers)

Residential care

The Laing and Buisson *Care of elderly people market survey 2000* found that, in 1999, 30 per cent of people in independent sector care homes were self-payers.

As the table below shows, the sources of funding for residential care have changed dramatically during the last 15 years. The percentage who are self-funded has decreased (though the actual numbers of people have increased, from 90,000 in 1986 to 116,000 in 1999, according to Laing and Buisson).

Table 3.26 Source of finance for residents in private and voluntary care homes for elderly and physically handicapped people, Great Britain 1986–1999, in percentages

Source	1986	1988	1990	1991	1992	1993	1994	1995	1996	1997	1998	1999
Self-pay	52	43	41	34	29	31	27	30	29	27	28	30
Preserved rights	44	54	56	63	66	65	50	35	28	20	16	12
Local authority	3	3	2	3	3	3	20	30	39	49	52	53
NHS funded	1	1	1	1	1	2	3	3	4	4	5	5
All sources (in thousands)	174	239	280	310	340	361	376	384	385	382	379	381

Source: Laing and Buisson (2000). *Care of elderly people market survey 2000*, p. 132

The PSSRU residential survey (1996) collected information on the average weekly charges for self-funders in residential and nursing homes (Table 3.27).

Table 3.27 Average weekly charges for self-funders

Location	Average charge for self-funders in residential homes (£)	Average charge in residential homes with a majority of self-funders (£)	Average charge for self-funders in nursing homes (£)
London boroughs	300	314	443
Other areas	234	232	332
London as % of other areas	128	135	133

Source: Netten *et al.* (1999)

The MEOC (1997) survey of residential care providers found that the mean price per week charged to self-funded residents was higher than the price for those whose care was funded through a contract with the local authority. This suggests there is some degree of cross-subsidisation from the clients who fund their own care to the local authorities.

Table 3.28 Prices per week by funding source, sample average

	Self-funded residents	Residents funded under contract with the homes' own local authority
Mean (£)	270.41	262.10
Number of providers	21	12

Source: MEOC (1999)

Home care

The MEOC study of domiciliary care providers in the independent sector also collected information on the hourly prices charged to privately funded clients.

Table 3.29 Hourly daytime prices for practical and personal care for privately funded clients (£/hour)

Region	Practical care				Personal care		
	Time of care	Mean	Minimum	Maximum	Mean	Minimum	Maximum
London and the South	Weekday	7.35	3.90	12.75	7.97	5.00	12.75
	Weekend	8.80	5.20	18.75	9.25	5.50	18.75
The North	Weekday	6.58	4.00	11.00	6.67	4.25	11.00
	Weekend	7.30	4.50	11.00	7.39	4.50	11.00

Source: Matosevic *et al.* (2001)

In contrast to the findings for residential care prices, the study found that the range of prices and the average charge for practical and personal care was generally lower for privately funded clients than for publicly funded clients.

4   Remuneration and terms and conditions of employment of care and support workers

The QLFS provides data on the gross hourly rate of pay in the UK. The data presented here are from four pooled quarters during 1998 (Winter 1997 to Autumn 1998). The National Minimum Wage came into force in April 1999 and it is currently set at £3.70 for people over 22 (rising to £4.10 from October 2001) and £3.20 for people aged 18–22 (Department of Trade and Industry (DTI) web page: www.dti.gov.uk). The data shown here were collected prior to the introduction of the minimum wage. Even for occupations where the mean hourly pay is above the minimum wage, mean rates of pay of these low-paid jobs are expected to have risen since the minimum wage was introduced.

Table 4.1 shows the occupations that, with 95 per cent statistical confidence, share the same gross hourly mean salary as care assistants. This would show the alternatives that care assistants would have if they wanted to change jobs but still earn the same salary. Whereas most care assistants are women, some of the occupations listed below tend to employ less women, or might require sets of skills that would not make them a real alternative. The MEOC study suggests that the single occupation that care assistants are most often thought to consider as an alternative is retail, especially 'stacking shelves' in local supermarkets.

Table 4.1 Occupations that share the same mean gross hourly pay as care assistants, using the 95% confidence interval around the means

Occupation	Mean salary	95% Confidence interval	Median
Shelf fillers	4.38	4.18,4.58	4.14
Domestic, housekeepers, etc.	4.41	3.98,4.83	4.04
Housekeepers (non-domestic)	4.42	4.06,4.77	4.02
Clergy	4.55	4.55,5.74	4.77
Chefs, cooks	4.55	4.37,4.72	4.16
Care assistants	**4.57**	**4.48,4.67**	**4.26**
Packers, bottlers, etc.	4.57	4.42,4.71	4.21
Farm workers	4.59	4.18,5.01	4.47
Cab drivers and chauffeurs	4.61	4.20,5.02	4.13
Rounds and van salespersons	4.71	4.19,5.24	4.72
Hospital porters	4.72	4.38,5.06	4.43
Publicans, club stewards	4.74	4.30,5.19	4.39
Bakery etc process operatives	4.85	4.54,5.17	4.50
Messengers, couriers	4.87	3.95,5.79	4.00
Reception telephonists	4.91	4.61,5.22	4.79
Horticultural trades	4.97	3.96,5.98	4.17
Butchers, meat cutters	4.98	4.61,5.34	4.90
Making, processing labourers	5.06	4.60,5.51	4.84
Weighers, graders, sorters	5.23	4.44,6.03	4.45

Source: Based on Almond and Kendal (2000), using the QLFS

Note: Occupations for which there were less than 50 observations have been excluded

Residential care

Table 4.2 shows the basic hourly wage rates in six-hourly wage bands reported in a survey of residential accommodation for elderly people (Netten *et al.*, 1999). The table shows that, in 1996, the majority of nursing homes and private residential homes were paying basic wage rates below £4.00 per hour, compared to almost 90 per cent of local authority homes which were paying rates in the £4.00–£5.00/hour wage band.

Table 4.2 Basic hourly wage rates: percentage in each hourly wage band, by home type

Amount (£)	Nursing	Private residential	Voluntary residential	Dual registered	Local authority	All
£2 to < £3	13.9	20.3	1.6	9.5	0	8.7
£3 to <£4	85.5	78.2	53.5	71.4	3.1	52.6
£4 to <£5	12.1	6.8	38.6	14.3	88.1	34.6
£5 to <£6	0.6	0.8	6.3	4.8	6.9	3.6
£6 to <£7	0	0	0	0	1.26	0.3
£7 to <£8	0	0.8	0	0	0.6	0.3
Total	**165**	**133**	**127**	**42**	**159**	**647**

Source: Netten *et al.* (1999)

Home care

The Laing and Buisson (2000) survey of independent sector home care workers found that for-profit providers typically paid domiciliary care workers premiums of £0.50–£0.60 per hour for weekend working, whereas not-for-profit providers offered more generous premiums of £1.00 per hour or more for weekend working (Table 4.3).

Table 4.3 Average pay for hourly paid home care workers by trading status

Trading basis	Weekday £ per hour		Weekend £ per hour	
	personal care	practical care	personal care	practical care
Sole trader	£4.00	£3.90	£4.60	£4.40
Limited company	£4.20	£3.90	£4.80	£4.50
Voluntary organisation	£4.40	£4.40	£5.70	£5.30
All provider sectors	£ 4.20	£4.00	£4.90	£4.60

Source: Laing and Buisson (2000). *Domiciliary Care Markets 2000*

5   Staff turnover

There is a high turnover of staff in the care and support sector, and this section explores this in greater detail.

5.1 Vacancy and turnover rates for different types of support workers

The recruitment and retention survey (Social and Health Care Workforce Group, 2000b) collected data from 83 SSDs in England (56 per cent of SSDs), and from a sample of 1,000 independent sector residential and nursing homes (of which 241, i.e. 19 per cent, responded). The vacancy rate is calculated as the number of vacancies as a percentage of the total number of positions. The turnover rate is calculated as the number of leavers as a percentage of the numbers employed.

Table 5.1 Vacancy and turnover rates for different types of support workers, local authority staff, England, 2000

Vacancy and turnover	Field social care worker	Home care worker	Residential LA					
			Manager/supervisor			Care staff		
			Child	OP	Other adults	Child	OP	Other adults
Vacancy rate (%)	16.0	11.3	4.6	5.9	6.9	11.9	9.4	11.5
Turnover rate (%)	15.3	16.0	8.0	6.8	8.8	10.5	11.0	12.3

Source: SHCWG (2000b)

Note: Field social care worker include team leaders/managers. Home care workers include home care staff/home helps.

Table 5.2 Vacancy and turnover rates for independent sector residential and nursing homes, England, 2000

	Manager/supervisor	Care staff
Vacancy rate (%)	5.2	9.3
Turnover rate (%)	13.1	21.8

Source: SHCWG (2000b)

5.2 Differences in vacancy and turnover rates for statutory and independent sector employers

It is evident that high turnover is a feature of social care employment, but this is even more of a feature of the independent sector than of local authority employment.

Table 5.3 Vacancy rate (%)

Home type	Residential local authority					
	Manager/supervisor			Care staff		
	Child	OP	Other adults	Child	OP	Other adults
Local authority homes	4.6	5.9	6.9	11.9	9.4	11.5
Independent	6.8	4.5	3.5	8.5	9.8	10.5

Source: SHCWG (2000b)

Table 5.4 Turnover rate (%)

Home type	Residential local authority					
	Manager/supervisor			Care staff		
	Child	OP	Other adults	Child	OP	Other adults
Local authority homes	8.0	6.8	8.8	10.5	11.0	12.3
Independent	21.0	9.7	13.5	21.9	25.8	15.2

Source: SHCWG (2000b)

5.3 Differences in vacancy and turnover rates for different geographical areas?

Tables 5.5 and 5.6 show that the vacancy rates for London and the South East tend to be higher than those in other areas. The geographical differences for turnover rates (Tables 5.7 and 5.8) are less clear, as they are rather different for each type of support worker.

Table 5.5 Vacancy rates (as a percentage) for different types of support workers, local authority staff, England, 2000, by region

Region	Field social care worker	Home care worker	Residential local authority					
			Manager/supervisor			Care staff		
			Child	OP	Other adults	Child	OP	Other adults
London	19.9	20.3	6.1	4.7	14.1	14.4	12.8	8.7
SE/East	19.8	8.9	8.6	11.5	3.2	13.8	14.1	18.4
Midlands/ SW	13.0	9.0	12.2	5.4	4.2	12.3	6.3	8.5
North	14.0	10.0	6.1	4.0	7.4	10.0	8.1	10.5
England	16.0	11.3	4.6	5.9	6.9	11.9	9.4	11.5

Source: SHCWG (2000b)

Table 5.6 Vacancy rate (%). Independent sector residential and nursing homes, England, 2000, by region

Region	Manager/supervisor	Care staff
London	4.9	15.0
SE/East	3.5	11.0
Midlands/ SW	5.0	4.8
North	4.9	8.9
England	5.2	9.3

Source: SHCWG (2000b).

Table 5.7 Turnover rates (as a percentage) for different types of support workers, local authority staff, England, 2000, by region

Region	Field social care worker	Home care worker	Residential local authority					
			Manager/supervisor			Care staff		
			Child	OP	Other adults	Child	OP	Other adults
London	21.9	16.5	3.2	9.0	13.8	11.1	13.8	11.8
SE/East	13.3	21.7	8.8	9.4	13.7	7.7	10.8	15.4
Midlands/ SW	14.9	17.1	12.1	4.2	7.9	13.5	10.3	14.6
North	13.1	13.7	7.9	6.5	6.3	9.6	10.4	10.6
England	15.3	16.0	8.0	6.8	8.8	10.5	11.0	12.3

Source: SHCWG (2000b).

Table 5.8 Turnover rate (%) for independent sector residential and nursing homes, England, 2000

Region	Manager/supervisor	Care staff
London	10.0	22.9
SE/East	10.8	23.8
Midlands/SW	10.5	15.6
North	24.6	25.9
England	13.1	21.8

Source: SHCWG (2000b).

5.4 Recruitment difficulties

The UKHCA Survey (Mathew, 2000) found that over three-quarters of providers had reported difficulties in recruiting home care workers and that providers in the South East were most likely to find recruitment a problem.

Table 5.9 Percentage of providers experiencing difficulty with recruitment by region (n = 275)

Region	Percentage of providers
South West	76
South East	86
Midlands	66
North	68
All regions	76

Source: Mathew (2000)

5.5 Use of long-term agency workers

The Recruitment and Retention Survey (Social and Health Care Workforce Group, 2000b) also collected data on the use of long-term care agency workers in SSDs. It found that the majority of SSDs did use long-term care agency workers (Table 5.10). The survey also found that 'the reasons given by SSDs for using long-term agency workers emphasised cover for vacancies or absence, with very few indicating replacement of permanent posts' (SHCWG 2000b, p. 4).

Table 5.10 Use of long-term agency workers by SSDs, England, 2000

	London	SE/East	Midlands/ SW	North	Total (England)
SSDs using long-term agency workers	13	13	10	16	52
SSDs **not** using long-term agency workers	1	2	8	12	23

Source: SHCWG (2000b)

Note: Long-term agency workers are those in post for over a month.

6 Qualifications and training

Local authority staff

The 1999 Social Services Workforce Survey collected data on the qualifications that social services staff held and were studying for. Data were collected on all qualifications held by staff, allowing for multiple recording, with the numbers holding more than one qualification also recorded. Table 6.1 shows that 36 per cent of all local authority staff were qualified. The most common qualification was professional social work held by two-thirds of all qualified staff. It is also striking that 93.5 per cent of home care staff lacked formal qualifications.

Table 6.1 Qualifications held by social services staff (1997–99), in percentages

Qualifications	Area (a)	Area (b)	Home care	Day care	Resid. care	Special . needs	**Total**
Professional social work	37.3	95	0.3	7.1	6.2	24.0	**22.9**
Management (incl. NVQ assessor)	2.9	14.7	1.7	5.1	4.7	6.2	**5.7**
Nursing	0.9	0.0	0.9	2.0	2.2	3.2	**1.2**
S/NVQ	6.7	0.0	3.2	10.1	6.6	4.4	**4.6**
Other	13.6	0.0	1.7	13.5	12.4	19.0	**6.5**
Total qualified	56.5	95.0	6.5	42.5	26.4	47.2	**36.4**
Total not qualified	43.5	5.0	93.5	57.5	73.6	52.8	**63.6**
Numbers in the sample	6,120	45,217	78,571	31,676	63,967	1,502	**222,053**

Source: SHCWG (2000a)

Area (a): covers OT, OT assistants and community workers; Area (b): senior directing staff, assistant directors, team leaders, assistant team leaders, and field social workers and care managers.

The figures in the next table show that 12 per cent of all social services staff were studying for qualifications. This was highest in residential settings (17.8 per cent), followed by day care (14.6 per cent), specialist needs establishments (12.9 per cent), while the lowest proportions of staff studying for qualifications were found in domiciliary care (6.4 per cent).

The most commonly sought qualifications were S/NVQs (8.5 per cent of all staff, or 71 per cent of those studying), followed by management (2.2 per cent), professional social work (0.6 per cent) and other qualifications (0.9 per cent).

Table 6.2 Qualifications being studied for by social services staff (1997–1999), in percentages

Qualifications	Area (a)	Home care	Day care	Resid. care	Special needs	**Total**
Professional social work	5.1	0.0	0.5	0.8	2.1	**0.6**
Management (incl. NVQ Assessor)	0.8	1.2	2.7	3.4	2.0	**2.2**
Nursery nursing	N/A	N/A	0.1	N/A	N/A	**0.0**
Nursing	0.0	0.0	0.0	0.0	0.2	**0.0**
S/NVQ	3.9	4.8	10.3	12.7	6.2	**8.5**
Other	1.5	0.4	1.2	1.4	3.3	**0.9**
Total studying	10.8	6.4	14.6	17.8	12.9	**12.0**
Total not studying	89.2	93.6	85.4	82.2	87.1	**88.0**
Total studying for more than one	0.6	0.0	0.2	0.4	0.3	**0.2**
Total employment	100.0	100.0	100.0	100.0	100.0	**100.0**

Source: SHCWG (2000a)

Notes: Area (a) covers occupational therapists, OT assistants and community workers. Information on qualifications being studied for was not collected for the other area groups (Area (b)) presented in Table 6.5.
'Home care' covers home care organisers, assistant home care organises and home care staff/home helps.
'Day care' covers care staff in all day care settings except playgroups, nursery centres and community centres.
'Residential care' covers care staff in all residential settings.
'Specialist needs establishments' covers children's establishments.
The number of staff studying for 'other' qualifications may be slightly overestimated due to double counting of staff studying for more than one qualification.

Independent sector staff

Residential care

In all homes in England, in 1996, a total of 113,400 (31.6 per cent) of the staff were qualified. The most frequent qualifications held by staff were nursing qualifications (21.5 per cent), followed by NVQ qualifications held by 7.2 per cent of staff. Staff in nursing homes were more likely to be professionally qualified, as would be expected given the requirements of regulations.

Table 6.3 Qualifications (%) held by type of home in England, 1996

Type of home	Number of qualified staff	% of qualified staff
Residential and dual registered homes		
Nursing qualifications	32,400	13.5
NVQ assessor	10,100	4.2
NVQ	18,600	7.7
Social work	2,900	1.2
Other	17,500	7.3
Total	66,100	27.5
Nursing homes		
Nursing qualifications	44,700	37.5
NVQ assessor	5,700	4.8
NVQ	7,400	6.2
Social work	100	0.1
Other	2,100	1.8
Total	47,400	39.7
All homes		
Nursing qualifications	77,200	21.5
NVQ assessor	15,800	4.4
NVQ	26,000	7.2
Social work	3,000	0.8
Other	19,600	5.5
Total	**113,400**	**31.6**

Source: LGMB (1997)

A total of 51,750 (14.4 per cent) of the staff employed in residential and nursing homes were studying for qualifications. The figures in Table 6.4 show that 9 per cent of all staff were studying for NVQ.

Table 6.4 Staff studying for qualifications by qualification and type of home, England, 1996

	Number of qualified staff	Percentage of qualified staff
Residential and dual registered homes		
Nursing qualifications	1,300	0.5
NVQ assessor	4,720	2.0
NVQ (any level)	21,870	9.1
Social work	430	0.2
Other	7,570	3.2
Total	35,890	15.0
Nursing homes		
Nursing qualifications	2,390	2.0
NVQ assessor	1,790	1.5
NVQ (any level)	10,500	8.8
Other	1,190	1.0
Total	15,870	13.3
All homes		
Nursing qualifications	3,680	1.0
NVQ assessor	6,500	1.8
NVQ (any level)	32,370	9.0
Social work	430	0.1
Other	8,770	2.4
Total	**51,750**	**14.4**

Source: LGMB (1997)

Home care

Nearly one-third (31 per cent) of home care workers who responded to a UKHCA survey in 2000 held and/or were studying for a qualification. These figures are higher than those reported in Laing and Buisson's 1997 survey, in which only 15 per cent had a qualification.[7] More than half of workers had received training during the previous 12 months, and workers who had a qualification were more likely to have received recent training than those without.

Table 6.5 Percentage of home care workers with/or studying for a qualification

Qualification	% with qualifications	% studying for qualifications
Nursing qualifications	4.8	1.9
NVQ/SVQ 2/3/4/	8.5	8.3
Other social/health care qualifications, e.g. BTEC	4.7	0.9
Any relevant qualifications above and other qualifications	19.6	14.4
Total holding and/or studying for qualifications	31.0	

Source: Mathew (2000)

The UKHCA study also found a marked difference in the proportion of staff with qualifications by age group. It was found that younger (under 30 years) were much more likely to have qualifications than those in all subsequent age groups (Table 6.6).

Table 6.6 Proportion of workers holding relevant qualifications by age group

Qualifications	Age group of care worker				
	Under 30 years	30–39 years	40–49 years	50 years and over	All ages
Nursing qualifications	2	3	5	8	5
NVQ qualifications	12	9	8	8	9
Other social care qualifications	14	5	2	1	5
Any qualification held	29	19	17	18	20
Base numbers	244	312	320	402	1,278

Source: Mathew (2000)

---

[7] A higher proportion of home care workers reported in the UKHCA survey may reflect a bias in their sample which was self-selecting.

A higher proportion of the independent sector home care workers in the sample are qualified than staff in local authority home care services. However, the comparison with the local authority sector must be treated with caution because it is not known whether respondents to the UKHCA survey are representative of independent sector home care workers.

Table 6.7 Percentage of *independent* sector and *local authority* home care workers holding qualifications

Qualifications	Percentage of local authority home care workers	Percentage of independent sector respondents to survey (n = 1292)
NVQ 2	1.8	8.2
NVQ 3	0.7	2.4
NVQ 4	0.1	0.5
Nursing	0.8	4.8
NVQ assessor	0.8	0.7

Source: SHCWG (2000a)

About one in five of the domiciliary care providers surveyed in the MEOC research reported that about half of their staff held a social care qualification (Table 6.8). A similar proportion (19 per cent) of providers indicated that most or all of their staff had such qualifications. However, the latter figures may overestimate the number of people with qualifications if set alongside figures from the Improvement and Development Agency, which suggest that only 7 per cent of local authority domiciliary care staff have a formal qualification and that only 6 per cent of staff are studying for qualifications (Social and Health Care Workforce Group, 1999).

Table 6.8 Proportion of home care workers with nursing or social care qualifications

Proportion	Nursing qualifications		Social care qualifications	
	Count	% of 155	Count	% of 155
None	52	33.5	20	12.9
Small proportion	68	43.9	71	45.8
About half	7	4.5	29	18.7
Most or all	2	1.3	30	19.4
Missing	26	16.8	5	3.2

Source: Matosevic *et al.* (2001)

The study found that over 90 per cent of respondents pay for unqualified staff to train for qualifications. Some 75 per cent of the interview sample did not receive any assistance from the local authority to provide training.

7   Household level data

This section describes the role of care workers in providing services to people living in their own homes, using household level data. It also addresses the extent to which the inputs of care workers can be seen as complementary to informal care.

The module of questions for people aged 65 years and over, which is included from time to time in the General Household Survey (GHS), provides data on their living circumstances, health, ability to perform a range of domestic and other tasks, and the use they make of health and social services (Bridgwood, 2000). Most of the data presented here come from analysis of the 1994–5 and 1998–9 GHS carried out for the PSSRU long-term care demand and finance model.

Table 7.1 Use of some personal social services by people aged 65 and over in the month before interview, 1991–8, Great Britain (percentages)

Type of service	1991	1994	1998
Home help (local authority)	9	8	4
Private domestic help	4	7	9
Meals-on-wheels	3	3	2
Day centre	3	3	3
District nurse/health visitor	6	6	5
Number in GHS sample	3,731	3,476	3,080

Source: Bridgwood (2000), Table 46, p. 60

The table shows that use of the local authority home help service has declined markedly since 1994, with a reduction in use from 8 per cent to 4 per cent. Use of private domestic help has increased from 7 per cent to 9 per cent since 1994.

Pickard *et al.* (2001) have explored in detail the receipt of services by people aged 65 or over in the 1994 and 1998 GHS. They have found that, between 1994 and 1998, there has been a decline in the use of some services and increases in the use of others, with different effects on different dependency groups. Table 7.2 shows the probability of receiving a service of any kind, including private domestic help, in 1994 and 1998.

Services include receipt of home help/care, district nursing, meals-on-wheels and private domestic help, and attendance at day centres and lunch clubs.

Table 7.2 Proportion receiving any formal service (including private domestic help) by dependency, 1994–5 and 1998–9

Level of dependency	1994–5		1998–9	
	Total in group	Proportion receiving services	Total in group	Proportion receiving services
No dependency	2,489	11.6	2,233	10.7
Slight dependency (IADL problems only)	244	37.3	234	38.5
Moderate dependency (One ADL)	357	38.1	303	34.0
Severe dependency (two or more ADLs)	379	52.5	308	50.3
All in sample	3,469	20.6	3,078	19.1

Source: Pickard *et al.* (2001), from analysis of GHS, 1994–5 and 1998–9, population over 65 years, Great Britain

In 1994, 56 per cent of all older people in the sample reported receipt of informal help (e.g. help provided by relatives, neighbours, friends) with domestic tasks. In 1998, the figure was 52 per cent. A very high proportion of people with dependency problems in both samples received informal help. In 1994, the proportion of all those with dependency who received informal care was 83 per cent, and in 1998 it was 81 per cent. Table 7.3 below compares the probability of receiving services, between those who receive informal care and those who do not. The proportion of people receiving services between 1994 and 1998 has declined both for those in receipt of informal help and for those not in receipt of informal help, but the change overall has been small.

Table 7.3 Probability of receiving services by receipt of informal help with domestic tasks, 1994–5 and 1998–9

Dependency	In receipt of informal help		Not in receipt of informal help	
	1994–5	1998–9	1994–5	1998–9
Non dependent	11	12	12	11
All with dependency	39	36	64	62
All	23	22	18	16
Number in sample	1,950	1,605	1,519	1,464

Source: Pickard *et al.* (2001) from analysis of the GHS, 1994–5 and 1998–9, population over 65, Great Britain

Note: Services include home care, private domestic help, district nurse, day centre, meals-on-wheels and lunch club.

Table 7.4 examines the total number of visits by 'formal services' to people (allowing both coverage and intensity to be taken into account) and distribution between those with and without informal help. Overall, more than half of all formal services are provided to people who have informal help. This table shows that, to some extent, formal services act as a complement to informal care.

Table 7.4 Proportion of all visits by each service to people, with and without informal help with domestic tasks, 1998–9

Type of service	% of total visits to people with informal help	% of total visits to people without informal help
Home care	60	40
Private domestic help	49	51
District nurse	68	32
Day centre	67	33
Meals-on-wheels	58	42
Lunch club	58	42
Visits from all services	58	42
Total number of people	1,605 (52%)	1,464 (48%)

Source: Pickard *et al.* (2001) from analysis of the GHS 1998–9, population over 65, Great Britain

References

Almond S, Kendall J. *Low pay in the UK: the case for a three sector comparative approach.* Civil Society Working Paper 6. London: London School of Economics and Political Science, 2000.

Audit Commission. *Charging with care: how councils charge for home care.* London: Audit Commission, 2000.

Bridgwood A. *People aged 65 and over.* London: Office for National Statistics, Government Statistical Service, 2000.

Department of Health. *Modernising social services: promoting independence, improving protection, raising standards.* Cm 4169. London: The Stationery Office, 1998, para. 5.1.

Department of Health. *NHS hospital and community health services non-medical staff in England: 1999–2000.* Bulletin 2001/3. London: Office for National Statistics, Government Statistical Service, 2001.

Department of Health. *Personal social services staff of social service departments at 30 September 1999 England.* Bulletin 2000/6. London: Office for National Statistics, Government Statistical Service, 2000a.

Department of Health. *Personal social services current expenditure in England: 1998–99.* Statistical Bulletin 2000/10. London: Office for National Statistics, Government Statistical Service, 2000b.

Department of Health. *Local authority staffing statistics.* 2001; http://www.doh.gov.uk/public/psstaff.htm.

Department of Health. *Personal social services current expenditure in England.* 2001; http://www.doh.gov.uk/public/pss_stat.htm.

Laing and Buisson. *Care of elderly people market survey 2000.* London: Laing and Buisson Publications, 2000.

Laing and Buisson. *Domiciliary care markets 2000.* London: Laing and Buisson Publications, 2000.

Laing and Buisson. *Healthcare market review 1999–2000.* London: Laing and Buisson Publications, 2000.

Lewis H, Fletcher P, Hardy B, Milne A, Waddington E. *Promoting well-being: developing a preventive approach with older people.* Oxford: Anchor Trust, 1999.

Local Government Management Board (LGMB) and the Association of Directors of Social Services (ADSS). *Social services workforce analysis 1997. Main report.* Social services workforce series. Report no. 24. London: LGMB/ADSS, 1998.

Local Government Management Board. *Independent sector workforce survey 1996. Residential and nursing homes in Great Britain.* London: LGMB, 1997.

Mathew D. *Who cares? a profile of the independent sector home care workforce in England.* United Kingdom Home Care Association, 2000.

Matosevic T, Knapp M, Kendall J, Forder J, Ware P, Hardy B. *Domiciliary care providers in the independent sector.* PSSRU Monograph forthcoming, 2001.

Mixed Economy of Care Research (MEOC) team. *Residential care provider study.* Unpublished report to the Department of Health, 1999.

Netten A, Bebbington A, Darton R, Forder J, Myles K. *1996 survey of care homes for elderly people. Final report.* Discussion paper 1423/2. Canterbury: Personal Social Services Research Unit, University of Kent, 1999.

Pickard L, Wittenberg R, Comas-Herrera A, Davies B, Darton R. Relying on informal care in the new century? Informal care for elderly people in England to 2031. *Ageing and Society* 2000; 20: 745–72.

Pickard L, *et al.* Work in progress at PSSRU. 2001.

Quilgars D. *Low intensity support services.* Bristol: The Policy Press and the Joseph Rowntree Foundation, 2000.

Registered social landlords. *Insight.* Housing Corporation, London: Housing Corporation, 1999.

Social and Health Care Workforce Group. *Social services workforce analysis 1998. Main report.* Social Services Workforce Series. Report no. 26. London: Employment Surveys and Research Unit, Employers Organisation, 1999.

Social and Health Care Workforce Group. *Social services workforce analysis 1999. Main report.* Social Services Workforce Series. Report no. 28. London: Employment Surveys and Research Unit, Employers Organisation, 2000a; http://www.lg-employers.gov.uk/documents/esru/sswmain99.pdf.

Social and Health Care Workforce Group. *Social services recruitment and retention survey 2000. Summary of findings.* London: Employment Surveys and Research Unit, Employers Organisation, 2000b.

Ware P, Matosevic T, Forder J, Hardy B, Kendall J, Knapp M, Wistow G. *Movement and change: independent sector domiciliary care providers between 1995 and 1999.* Leeds: Nuffield Institute for Health, University of Leeds, 2001.

Wittenberg R, Pickard L, Comas-Herrera A, Davies B, Darton R. Demand for long-term care for elderly people in England to 2031. *Health Statistics Quarterly* 2001; in press.

Wittenberg R, Pickard L, Comas-Herrera A, Davies B, Darton R. *Demand for long-term care: projections of long-term care finance for elderly people.* Canterbury: Personal Social Services Research Unit, University of Kent, Canterbury, 1998.

Appendix 2

Consultation with service users and carers

In addition to the written material submitted to the Inquiry, and a series of meetings with various 'witnesses', we also arranged a number of consultative meetings with groups of service users and carers. The purpose of these meetings was to hear the voices of people at first hand, and to ensure that attention was paid to perspectives that might have been excluded from the more formal evidence collection.

Meetings were arranged with the help of:

- Better Government for Older People (Older People's Advisory Group)
- Shaping Our Lives (National User Group)
- Service users contacted through projects of the National Schizophrenia Fellowship
- Trustees of Carers National Association.

In all, more than 60 people were involved in the consultation meetings, and we are extremely grateful to all those who participated.

A note summarising the key findings from the consultation is included in this appendix. An earlier version of this was shared with all participants in the meetings, and was positively received.

King's Fund Care and Support Inquiry Feedback on Key Themes and Issues from User Consultation

The King's Fund Care and Support Inquiry into the quality of services in health, housing and social care settings arranged a number of meetings to consult with people who have first hand experience of using services. The purpose of the consultation was threefold:

- to identify problems in the quality of care and support services, and the reasons for these
- to identify the characteristics of good services, and to highlight good practice
- to make recommendations on what would make the most difference.

This feedback note draws on the findings from five consultation meetings which took place in January to February 2001. In total, more than 60 people were involved in these meetings.

Problems and concerns over services

A number of key themes recurred in all the meetings, including:

- ☹ poor attitudes of some staff
- ☹ hurried delivery of service
- ☹ lack of humanity and compassion
- ☹ poor quality of some staff
- ☹ shortcomings in training
- ☹ no continuity of care
- ☹ confusion over accountability

- ☹ services that don't meet needs and which are insensitive to cultural diversity
- ☹ a minority of staff are abusive, and examples exist of physical, sexual and psychological abuse of service users.

Service users often had considerable understanding of how demanding it is to be a care worker, and saw this as an explanation for some of the problems in service quality:

Care staff need to earn a living! The question of how much people are paid is crucial.

However, it was also believed that poor quality of some staff reflected broader recruitment issues:

A problem when you are relying on people who can't get a job anywhere else.

A lack of compassion on the part of a minority of staff was identified by many service users:

They need to treat us as human beings, not as lumps of meat.

People who were users of mental health services (especially hospital-based services) were more likely than others to report staff treating them with a lack of respect or with aggression, and to lack empathy:

I don't understand why these people go into this work, because they don't care.

Some staff can be highly controlling, and some users of mental health services were concerned about how drugs could be used as an explicit means of controlling people:

They just want to quieten you down all the time – any trouble and they bang in the drugs.

Equally, the use of sectioning powers (or the threat of it) was felt to be used as an explicit sanction, as was the withdrawal of services and support from people who were challenging for services (*if people are a bit difficult, they are not tolerated*). These experiences were not unique to mental health service users; another person with a fluctuating chronic illness described a similar experience:

I've been psychologically abused and bullied with the threat that if I don't toe the line I will lose service support.

Poor awareness of the significance of cultural diversity was also identified by service users from black and minority ethnic communities. For example, one user of mental health services commented:

No one ever talked to me about my race and background in all of this, and yet that was central to me and my experience.

Other people pointed out that even when staff went into caring work for what they might think were the best of motives, these were often considerably different from what service users

would see as centrally important, for example:

People go into these professions to come and 'look after' you. It isn't about empowerment and enabling people to live independent lives – there are major training issues there. And you have to fight for your rights all the time and struggle against that culture.

At the same time, there was some recognition that the low status and position of many care staff was itself an obstacle:

Workers can't empower service users unless they themselves are empowered.

Genuine user involvement can be an important dimension of empowerment. For some people, the experience of involvement in planning has been tokenistic and patronising, and they have been denied full participation. Others have emphasised the vital contribution that service users can make in monitoring service quality, for example:

Professionals don't know the tell-tale signs to look for, and services are good at hiding things; you need to have service users going in to services and picking up signs of things that are wrong.

Others also emphasised that user monitoring of services is vital in giving other users a voice, because people will talk more openly to fellow service users than to professionals.

The hurried way in which services are often delivered was a recurring complaint.

People haven't got time to spend with you because their case-loads are so intense.

It was also recognised that time pressures arose because services were covering large geographical areas and were not using local staff. The need to travel between clients greatly reduced the actual contact time available, with service users often feeling that they are having to pay for a service they are not receiving:

You pay for an hour, and you get ten minutes!

The pressure for greater efficiency in service delivery was also sometimes experienced negatively. Some service users described how an unpopular rationalisation of the 'meals-on-wheels service' had led to fortnightly deliveries of frozen meals, taking away the opportunity for daily human contact (however hurried).

These pressures on services were also seen by some service users in reduced time available to care workers to spend in interacting with clients during visits:

Staff are paid to do a job, and unless communication or interaction is designated as part of that job, then it doesn't get done.

The particular needs of residents of care homes were identified. There were concerns about the situation of people who were accommodated with others who had high levels of confusion that they did not share. In consequence, these frail elderly people were wholly isolated in an environment where there was no one they could communicate with, and where they were simply overlooked by staff.

The physical standards of care in hospitals was also identified as a matter of concern. Basic standards were frequently identified as poor, with shortages of bedding, lack of hot food (and lack of care for people needing help with feeding), and lack of attention to toileting needs.

The lack of continuity of care – with new care workers coming along all the time – was a further source of discontent. It was recognised that high turnover of staff contributed to the problem, which was also evident in care staff simply not turning up when they were expected (or not at all).

Most care and support services are provided through the independent sector, even though they may be commissioned by the local authority social services department. However, this separation of purchasing and provider roles can be hugely confusing for service users, who are left not knowing 'who is in charge':

What do you do with contracted staff? Who do you contact when things go wrong? There are repeated problems with staff who don't come when they are supposed to.

Knowing what to do, and finding a way through the system was frequently described as 'hard work':

You always need to make four or five phone calls even to find the person you need to speak to.

Characteristics of good services

The picture that was painted by service users and carers was by no means one of unremitting gloom. Indeed, the characteristics of good services, and the qualities of particular staff, were highlighted in all the consultations. The positive dimensions included:

☺ caring, reliable and friendly staff

☺ services that are pleasant to visit

☺ services that enhance confidence and self-esteem

☺ services that can put you in touch with other help.

Some innovative services for people with mental health needs (under the auspices of NSF) were experienced far more favourably than traditional services. The service premises were pleasant and were not viewed as stigmatising (they were not labelled like other services, and were places that people could walk into without feeling conspicuous). Compared with other services, these were *a godsend*.

An employment project that helped people into training opportunities and into employment was especially valued for the self-esteem that it helped service users to reclaim:

Having a job is the biggest thing in giving you respect, dignity, identity and self-worth.

What would make a difference?

Service users and carers had many suggestions on what needed to change. However, the major themes that were identified were the following:

- ensure staff are properly trained and qualified
- the role of care staff must be upgraded and enhanced with proper pay for the work they do
- involve service users in training of staff
- develop more innovative service models, and develop local solutions
- promote user involvement in services
- recognise that quality services cost money
- managers need more hands-on experience
- the role of care staff requires new 'super carers' – flexible, multi-skilled, and holistic
- scope for engaging volunteers in support, but without exploiting them.

Appendix 3

Individuals and organisations who made written or verbal submissions to the Inquiry, or were involved in consultation

Action on Elder Abuse, Jenkins, Ginny, Chief Executive.

Alcohol Concern, Boon, Sue, Assistant Director.

Alcohol Problems Advisory Service (APAS), de Vekey, Meriel, Policy Development Officer.

Anchor Trust, Belcher, John, Chief Executive.

Archway Centre, Walsall (National Schizophrenia Fellowship, NSF).

Association for Residential Care, Furze, Yvonne, National Branch Development Manager.

Association of Directors of Social Services (ADSS).

Audit Commission, Bolton, John, Director, Joint Reviews.

Barnet and Chase Farm Hospitals NHS Trust, Price, Miriam, Head of Professional Education and Training.

Best, Richard, Carer.

Better Government for Older People, Older People's Advisory Group.

Blackburn Social Services, Duxbury, Royce, Team Manager, Mental Health Support Services.

Body Positive.

British Association of Domiciliary Care (BADCO), Thompson, Valerie, and McAvoy, Roberta.

British Federation of Care Home Proprietors, Burns, Marion, Director.

Burton, John, Independent Social Care Consultant.

Capital Carers, Ward, Sue, Director.

Carers Centre, Oxford, Pugh, Katy, Manager.

Carers Impact, the King's Fund, Banks, Penny.

Carers National Association.

Caring Concern, Price, Carole, Care Manager.

Clear-A-Head, Employment Project, Romford (NSF).

Community Mental Health Directorate, Sheffield, Huws, Dr Rhodri.

Community Rehabilitation Team Network, Shield, Fiona, CRT Network Co-ordinator.

Consumers Association.

Dementia Services Development Centre, University of Stirling.

Department for Education and Employment.

Department of Health.

Down's Syndrome Association.

Exeter and District Learning Disability Service Abuse Group.

Extra Care, Belfast, McGinn, J, Quality Standards Manager.

First Community Health NHS Trust, Stafford. Corry, Sandra, Service Co-ordinator.

Further Education Funding Council, Vaughan Huxley, Merillie.

General Medical Council.

George House Trust.

Greater London Forum for the Elderly, Newman, Carole, Director.

Grinstead, Paul, Care Assistant.

Health Which, Gitter, Louise, Principal Researcher.

Home Farm Trust, Madden, Phil, Director of Service Development.

Hudson, John R, Independent Management and Information Technology Consultant.

Independent Healthcare Association. Taber, Sally, Head of Operational Policy; Blackburn, Sharon; Gunson, Elaine; Galipet, Michelle.

Initiatives in Care, Bell, Lesley.

Islington Chinese Association, Ng, Dr Stephen, Elderly Work Co-ordinator.

Jewish Care, Weinstein, Jenny, Quality Assurance Manager.

Keddie, Sue, Care Assistant.

Kent County Council, Huntingford, Pat, Head of Service Policy and Standards.

Kettering General Hospital NHS Trust, Mellon, Kim, Occupational Standards Trainer.

Kids Company, Holmes, Carol.

King's Fund.

Kingwood Trust. McGuire, Mary, Chief Executive.

Leeds Joint Planning, Ingram, Ruth, Adult Protection Co-ordinator.

Leonard Cheshire, Dutton, Bryan, Director General.

Liverpool Social Services Directorate, Bannister, Ann, Team Manager, Adult Protection Unit.

London Borough of Westminster, Social Services.

Marie Curie Cancer Care, Garland, Eva, Director of Nursing.

Mental Health Foundation, Duerdoth, Nigel, Director of Programmes.

Mushkil Aasaan.

National Association of Inspection and Registration Officers, Jefferson, Alan, Chair.

National Heads of Inspection and Registration.

National Institute for Social Work.

National Schizophrenia Fellowship (NSF).

Network Housing Association, Gunn, Alan, Manager, Housing Support Work.

NHS Executive.

North Mersey Community NHS Trust, Vose, Colin, Mental Health Education and Training Strategy Co-ordinator.

Nuffield Institute for Health, University of Leeds.

OutReach, Orton, Morwenna, Outreach Service Development Manager.

Parkinson's Disease Society, Meadowcroft, Robert, Director, Policy, Research and Information.

Patients Association.

Personal Social Services Research Unit (PSSRU), at London School of Economics and Political Science.

Portsmouth City Council, Manley, Gill, Training and Development Officer, Social Services.

Portsmouth Healthcare NHS Trust, Kanagaratnam, Dr S, Consultant Psychiatrist, Learning Disability.

Progressive Supranuclear Palsy (PSP) Association, Koe, Brigadier, Sir Michael, Chief Executive.

Rayner, Claire, Agony Aunt and Journalist.

RCN Learning Disability Forum, University of Manchester, Anderton, Paul.

Richardson, D, W and Richardson, E, Carers.

Royal Borough of Kingston Upon Thames, Social Services.

Royal College of Nursing, Hancock, Christine, General Secretary.

Royal College of Physicians, Alberti, Professor, Sir George, President.

Royal College of Psychiatrists, Fairbairn, Dr Andrew.

Royal College of Speech and Language Therapists, Pigram, Jenny, Deputy Head, Department of Education and Professional Development.

Royal Free Hospital, Morris, Dr Jackie, Consultant Physician.

Royal National Institute for the Deaf (RNID), Loosemore-Reppen, Gerda, Policy and Research Officer.

Royal Surgical Aid Society (RSAS Agecare).

Shaping Our Lives.

Sheffield NHS Community Trust.

Somerset Health Authority.

Stonham Housing with Care, Nelson, Liz, Quality Development Officer, Care and Support.

Stroke Association, Goose, Margaret, Chief Executive.

Surrey Oaklands NHS Trust, Kinsey, Peter.

Surrey Oaklands NHS Trust, Mental Health Team.

The Carers Centre, Oxford.

The Home Farm Trust, Madden, Phil, Director of Service Development.

The Housing Corporation.

The Kingwood Trust.

TOPSS England/UK.

Tower Hamlets Healthcare NHS Trust, Mattison, Vicky, Clinical Psychologist.

Tripod (Tri-Regional Interest and Project Group on Learning Disability), Thorpe, Liz.

Truttero, Suzanne, Carer.

Twigg, Dr Julia, University of Kent.

UNISON.

United Kingdom Central Council for Nursing, Midwifery and Health Visiting (UKCC), Williams, Margaret, Professional Officer, Community Nursing and Health Visiting.

United Kingdom Home Care Association (UKHCA), Mathew, Dinah, and McClimont, Bill.

University of Hull, Quest Service Development and Evaluation Team, Oakes, Dr Peter.

University of Manchester, Anderton, Paul, School of Nursing, Midwifery and Health Visiting.

University of Sheffield, School of Health and Related Research, Enderby, Pam, Professor, Chief of Community Rehabilitation.

West Berkshire Priority Care, Williams, Margaret, Patient Services Manager.

Wigan Social Services Department.